WILDERNESS
MEDICINE

Beyond First Aid

Fifth Edition

Help Us Keep This Guide Up to Date

Every effort has been made by the author and editors to make this guide as accurate and useful as possible. However, many things can change after a guide is published—new products and information become available, regulations change, techniques evolve, etc.

We would love to hear from you concerning your experience with this guide and how you feel it could be improved and be kept up to date. While we may not be able to respond to all comments and suggestions, we'll take them to heart and we'll also make certain to share them with the author. Please send your comments and suggestions to the following address:

The Globe Pequot Press
Reader Response/Editorial Department
P.O. Box 480
Guilford, CT 06437

Or you may e-mail us at:

editorial@globe-pequot.com

Thanks for your input.

WILDERNESS MEDICINE

Beyond First Aid

Fifth Edition

William W. Forgey, M.D.

The Globe Pequot Press

Guilford, Connecticut

This book is dedicated to my parents Gladys (Harmack) and Homer
Forgey, without whose continuous love and assistance none of this
would have been possible. And to my brother Jonathan and his wife
Florence, who round out the loving environment in which I was raised
and in which I live.

Cover photo: Photodisc
Cover and page design: Lisa Reneson

Library of Congress Cataloging-in-Publication Data
Forgey, William, W.
    Wilderness medicine: beyond first aid/William W. Forgey.—5th ed.
        p.   cm.
    ISBN 0-7627-0490-X
    1. Backpacking injuries. 2. Mountaineering injuries. 3. First aid in illness
and injury. I. Title.
RC88.9.H55F67   2000
616.02'52—dc21   99-39807
                                                                        CIP

Manufactured in the United States of America
Fifth Edition/SecondPrinting

Contents

Chapter 2: Body System Symptoms and Management, 27

Symptom Management, 27
Fever/Chills • Lethargy • Pain • Itch • Hiccups • Headache

Eye, 35
*Eye Patch and Bandaging Technique • Foreign Body Eye Injury
Contact Lenses • Eye Abrasion • Snow Blindness, or Ultraviolet
Conjunctivitis • Iritis • Allergic Conjunctivitis • Sties and Chalazia
Spontaneous Subconjunctival Hemorrhage • Blunt Trauma to the
Eye • Glaucoma*

Nose, 47
*Nasal Congestion • Foreign Body Nose Injury • Nose Bleed
Nose Fracture (Broken Nose)*

Ear, 49
*Earache • Outer Ear Infection • Middle Ear Infection • Foreign
Body Ear Injury • Ruptured Ear Drum • Temporal-Mandibular-
Joint (TMJ) Syndrome*

Mouth and Throat, 55
*Sore Throat • Infectious Mononucleosis • Mouth Sores • Gum
Pain or Swelling • Mouth Lacerations • Dental Pain • Lost
Filling • Loose or Dislodged Tooth • Pulling a Tooth*

Chest, 62
Pneumonia/Bronchitis • Pneumothorax • Pulmonary Embolus

Abdomen, 64
*Abdominal Pain • Vomiting • Motion Sickness • Diarrhea
Constipation • Hemorrhoids • Hernia • Bladder Infection*

Reproductive Organs, 74
*Venereal Diseases • Vaginal Discharge and Itching • Painful
Testicle • Menstrual Problems • Spontaneous Abortion • Ectopic
Pregnancy*

Poisoning, 79
*Plant or Food Poisoning • Petroleum Products Poisoning • Ciguatera
Poisoning • Scromboid Poisoning • Pufferfish Poisoning • Paralytic
Shellfish Poisoning*

Managing Diabetes, 81
Water and Waste, 82
*Oral Fluid Replacement Therapy • Water Purification • Human
Waste Disposal*

Preface

This edition marks the twentieth anniversary since the first publication of *Wilderness Medicine*. Recommended therapy in the first edition was based on a combination of field improvisation techniques and a modular first aid kit. The kit included multifunctional components to tailor it more readily to the nature of the trip being undertaken. Over the next several editions changes in medical theory and treatment were reflected and advocated, including the use of the initial, focused survey as an entry to treatment protocols; updates on infectious diseases; totally redesigned modular medical kit systems; and the incorporation of those medical technology advances in various disciplines that affected wilderness medicine.

Medicine and its components are hardly static. The effects of change ripple rapidly into outdoor medicine. Consequently, one advantage this book has over any other in this field is the use of my Web site, www.adventure-media.com/wilderness-medicine5/. At this location you can easily access color photographs and updated information concerning many subjects, such as: poisonous reptiles or plants, infectious disease risk maps, and further sources of information for cross-referencing. Information about relevant training programs and sources for obtaining the medical supplies discussed in the book are also included. The updates available on the Web site will allow this edition of the book to be kept as current as possible. Finally, direct e-mail links to me and the other authorities who have agreed to be part of the site make us easy to reach.

Be sure to check out www.adventure-media/wilderness-medicine5/ often. I'll look forward to hearing from you.

— William W. Forgey, M.D.
Crown Point, Indiana

Introduction

How to Use This Book

There are four ways to rapidly identify where to find the information you need.

First

A quick glance through the Contents can lead you to the proper chapter and subject.

Second

The Initial Survey (pages 10–11) and the Focused Survey (pages 11-12) not only describe how to perform a physical examination and what to look for, but these sections also refer you to the page of the book that tells you what to do about it!

Third

Throughout the book various sections have diagnostic tables with references to further evaluate or explain treatment options. For problems that fall into these categories, you can refer directly to these tables as indicated in the list below.

List of Diagnostic Tables/References

Fourth

The Clinical Reference Index, starting on page 238, provides a comprehensive cross-reference between symptoms, conditions, and treatments. Subjects are listed using both medical jargon and vernacular descriptions.

How to Prepare for Remote Wilderness Travel

Mental Preparation

How do you tell a guy you hate his guts because of the way he holds his fork?

Do not presume that medical problems will be the most significant challenges that you will encounter on a wilderness expedition. Instead they will be leadership and expedition behavior issues. Any breakdown in this area can, and does, lead to the most significant wilderness accidents—accidents that can easily magnify into serious medical disasters.

Most trip organizers are not able to take into account the psychology and social skills of all the participants, but if you can take such factors into consideration, you might avoid the stress and conflict that often turn a dream project into a nightmare. I have found that a ten-day preparatory trip is generally enough to identify idiosyncrasies that might indicate incompatibility.

The great outdoorsman Calvin Rutstrum once summed up this problem when he said to me one day, "How do you tell a guy you hate his guts by the way he holds his fork?" It's simply amazing how personal habits and quirks can grate on you. In reviewing many successful (and not so) relationships during stressful trips, I have come to the conclusion that the most favorable relationship is one of "respect"; it surpasses love, hate, fear, or any other human emotional form of interaction. If you truly respect a trip partner, you can tolerate mannerisms and faults that would otherwise be unacceptable.

Prepare yourself mentally to enjoy the trip. Be expecting both adversity and monotony on any long expedition. A wonderful publication that shows the insight necessary for this to succeed is *Paradise Creek* by David Scott, published by The Globe Pequot Press (also available at www.adventure-media.com/scott/). I believe this book epitomizes what a long expedition is all about. As I helped prepare and sponsor David and his partner, Scott Power, for their expedition to Paradise Creek, you'll even learn a little about me in there, too.

Plan a time schedule that allows for weather as well as terrain. Many accidents in the bush result from having to take chances while running out of time, food, etc., thus turning the expedition into a retreat—or worse, a retreat into a rout. The more shortages (in food, time, or other resources), the more resulting stress.

Physical Preparation

Proper pre-trip physical conditioning cannot be stressed too highly. While trying to survive exposure, a major factor is the ability to generate heat, which is directly related to the ability to produce work. This is achieved through physical conditioning as the limiting factor, not by how much food one consumes.

Obtain a pre-trip dental exam well in advance of the trip, thus allowing adequate time for possible needed corrections.

While a thorough physical examination is indicated for everyone, going to the extreme of cardiac stress testing (treadmill) is not required in persons without symptoms of chest pain. The exception would be the sedentary individual who was planning on significantly increasing the amount of exertion that he or she normally experienced.

Be certain that orthopedic deficiencies, other impairments, and allergies are addressed in the medical history. Be capable of coping with the identified deficiencies by adjusting trip plans or personnel.

The pre-trip physical should include attention to immunization schedules, which vary depending upon the region of the world to be visited (see Appendix B). As a minimum, each trip member should have had a tetanus booster within the previous ten years.

Make sure that everyone has had an eye examination within the previous three years. For those over forty, I recommend an eye exam (including glaucoma check) within the previous year. If significant vision impairment exists, carry spare glasses or contact lenses. Adequate eye protection, usually sunglasses, is a must for everyone.

Prepare an evacuation plan. Obtain adequate medical insurance, particularly if foreign travel is contemplated. And assemble a medical kit (Appendix A).

The Wilderness Expedition Medical Kit

The ideal medical kit will have multifunctional components to reduce the cost, bulk, weight, and simplify usage. It should also be modular to allow an increasing depth of care by including the more sophisticated modules only if the potential risks of the trip, or reduced access to medical help, warrants their inclusion. Cross-functional component versatility is also important. This means that the same problem can be treated with two or more kit components. This requires a minimal amount of medication, but provides depth in coverage when a particular item is consumed.

Most injuries and conditions described in this book can be treated with very little in the way of kit components. But I have included here state-of-the-art items that would provide ideal treatment. As this book has been written for those who may be isolated without ready access to professional medical care, the treatments discussed go beyond normal first aid. The kit described in Appendix A similarly goes beyond what would be considered a "first aid" kit. But the initial modules are indeed easily useable under first aid conditions. The kit consists of four units: Topical Bandaging Module, Non-Rx Oral Medication Module, Rx Oral/Topical Medication Module, and the Rx Injectable Medication Module.

As a minimum, the Topical Bandaging Module and Non-Rx Oral Medication Module will generally fulfill the vast majority of emergency treatment requirements. The Field Surgical Module and the prescription modules are designed for long-term, and more advanced patient care. All items listed in the kit modules can be obtained without a prescription, except in the modules clearly marked "Rx."

In addition to the above, everyone should carry a new piece of emergency equipment called "The Extractor." This four ounce plastic suction device is ideal for use in the first aid treatment of snake bite, puncture wounds, and venomous stings. It is far superior to the rubber suction cup snake bite kit. Note description of use on page 157.

Consideration must be given to a dental kit. Several are commercially available through backpacking and outdoor outfitters. As a minimum, a small bottle of oil of cloves can serve as a topical toothache treatment, see page 60.

A fever thermometer may be handy, but frankly, I never carry one. People wearing contact lenses should carry the special suction cup or rubber pincher device to aid in their removal. Consideration may be given to a stethoscope and blood pressure cuff, if you know how to use them. They are essential items for Search and Rescue Units, but not for the usual wilderness expedition.

Early pregnancy detection kits may have a role in long-term expeditions and in trekking or taking clients into wilderness areas. Such a kit is potentially useful when trying to determine the cause of severe lower abdominal pain in a female of child-bearing age, the concern being the possibility of a tubal pregnancy, which is a life-threatening emergency.

Provide an adequate means of water purification as indicated on page 83. Failing to do so can also be the cause of severe lower (and upper) abdominal pain. While I prefer the Katadyn water filtration system, water treatment can be as simple as bringing water to a boil.

Do I bring all of the items that I have listed in the Wilderness Expedition Medical Kit Modules in Appendix A? Yes! And no! It depends.

If I was hiking the Appalachian Trail I would carry a few pieces of Spenco 2nd Skin and tape, ibuprofen, Imodium, and possibly a decongestant. The rest of my load would be food and the other direct necessities of life, certainly not first aid items. For a three week canoe trip in Northern Canada with three other people, I would cut the quantities of the Appendix A kit drastically, but I would have representative items from each module along. For two of us spending six months in an isolated cabin or on a yacht in the Pacific, I would carry the Appendix A modules as written. Going with a team of a hundred assaulting a mountain, I'd add a lot more stuff. But the exact nature of that stuff would depend upon my assessment of the situation. This book and Appendix A give you a plan for the management of most remote area emergencies.

The more that you read on this subject and the more medical training that trip members receive, the better off everyone will be. I particularly recommend that you obtain a copy of *Medicine for the Backcountry* by Buck Tilton and Frank Hubbell, The Globe Pequot Press.

A frequent lament that I hear from prospective expedition members is that they do not know a physician who could help by writing prescriptions for an adequate expedition medical kit. It is for this reason that even the first edition of this book had an extensive nonprescription medical kit designed to handle most problems that one might encounter in the bush. A list of suppliers of the nonprescription medications and virtually all of the instruments and high tech bandaging material described in this book can be obtained by referring to links on my Web site at www.adventure-media.com/wilderness-medicine5/.

Improvisation

Be capable of improvising. Some of the joys of wilderness travel relate to being able to improvise and get along without some item that was lost or left at home.

Appendix A notes a variety of improvisational methods and/or objects to use when you do not have particular medications or items along. From the cook, the medic can borrow baking soda, salt, and sugar to manage profound diarrhea. The formula for making oral rehydration salt solution from these items is on page 83.

Vinegar, flour, and ammonia are useful in treating jellyfish tentacle attachments (page 169). Vinegar is also useful in treating sea urchin spine wounds (page 168) and sponge rash injuries (page 170).

Soap for cleaning wounds may also be obtained from the kitchen, if a surgical scrub is not carried in the medical kit. Granulated sugar sprinkled on abrasions is a field-expedient method of preventing infection when there are no antibiotics available.

Each fishing kit should have wire cutters, to remove a hook from people as well as fish. These wire cutters may also be used to destroy a zipper, sometimes a necessary project if anyone catches skin in the zipper mechanism.

Synthetic or wool clothing is needed to prevent and treat hypothermic conditions, especially a hat, socks, and shirts. Having adequate sleeping bags, and choosing those that twin, may prove life-saving in hypothermic conditions. It is surprising how many bags will twin, sometimes the foot of one to the head of the other. A full treatment of modern synthetic fabrics is provided in my book *Basic Essentials: Hypothermia* (The Globe Pequot Press).

Matches are a potential life-saver and should be available on every trip. I point out in the hypothermia book that a fire is a poor way of keeping warm; adequate clothing is instead the best solution for that problem. But building a giant fire is a method of getting warm in an emergency.

On extended trips a vitamin supplement might be appropriate in order to prevent deficiency syndromes, such as scurvy. There is no doubt that vitamin deficiencies ranked high among the reasons for death during the early days of polar exploration. We are not immune from them during the modern era either.

And for treating headaches, sometimes a cup of coffee is just the answer. Especially if the victim is having caffeine withdrawal.

One of the benefits of taking a wilderness first aid or wilderness first responder course is the amount of improvisation that they teach, particularly when it comes to splinting and bandaging techniques. A list of wilderness medical literature and course resources is listed on my Web site.

Chapter 1

Assessment and Stabilization

It's not what happens to you that matters, but how you react to it that counts.
—Epictetus, 1st Century A.D.

Assessment and Care

To aid the victim of sudden injury is similar to giving appropriate treatment to someone who complains of sickness or sudden pain from a non-injury cause. Proper care can only result if several basic steps are performed properly. The basics are straight forward. You should not be intimidated by this process. The problem with medicine in general is that there are so many possible diagnoses and treatments that the whole thing can seem overwhelming. It is really not, however, if you follow certain logical steps.

These logical steps form the basis of starting the decision tree that will lead almost automatically to a correct course of action. They simplify the process into a much less scary proposition. The initial phase is assessment; the second phase is treatment or stabilization. While the first aid approach only includes assessment, this book is concerned with developing approaches to definitive treatment that could be reasonably performed in remote areas by relatively untrained (and undoubtedly very concerned) friends of the suddenly impaired.

Trauma assessment is divided into two phases called the initial survey and focused survey. What good is a survey if you don't know what to do with the information? During rescue operations what you do with the information is to record it. This recorded information, which includes periodic reassessment data, can be valuable to physicians at treatment centers as it indicates either a stable patient or a deteriorating one and helps direct their future course of action. For those of us who are stuck with caring for the patient in a remote area, this data can be used to enter a decision tree that will help determine our best course of action. Sometimes this will be definitive treatment, other times it will amount to minimizing the damage and striving to keeping the victim as functional as possible or sometimes just alive.

Initial Survey

Survey the Scene

First: Before assessing the patient, assess the scene! Accidents tend to multiply. Make sure the scene is safe for the rescuers and the victim. Ensure that the situation does not become worse. This step can include such diverse aspects as avoiding further avalanche or rock falls to ensuring an adequate clothing and food supply for rescuers. Initially, however, scene assessment is to look for immediate hazards that

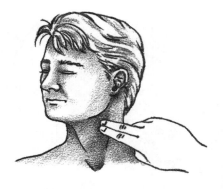

Figure 1–1: Position of fingers to check for the carotid artery pulse.

might result in more casualties among the group attempting to help the victim.

Check the Airway

Second: Check the airway. If the victim can talk, his airway is functioning. In an unconscious patient, place your ear next to his nose/mouth and your hand on his chest and look, listen, and feel for air movement.

No air movement: Check to see if the tongue is blocking the airway by pushing down on the forehead while lifting the chin. In case of possible neck injury, the airway can be opened with a lift of the jaw without movement of the neck.

Still no air movement: Pinch his nose and seal your mouth over his and try to force air into his lungs.

Still no air movement: Perform the Heimlich maneuver (page 18).

Once you are able to establish air movement, continue until the victim can take over on his own, see page 21.

Check Circulation

Check circulation by placing several of your fingertips lightly into the hollow below the angle of the patient's jaw. See Figure 1–1.

No pulse: Start CPR, see page 19.

Check Severe Bleeding

Check quickly for severe blood loss. Check visually and with your hands. Slide your hand under the victim to ensure that blood is not leaking into the ground or snow and check inside bulky garments for hidden blood loss.

Severe bleeding: Use direct pressure, see page 90.

Check the Cervical Spine

During the primary survey keep the head and neck as still as possible if there is any suspicion of a cervical spine injury. This may certainly be the case if the patient is unconscious or suffering from an accident such as a steep fall, a sudden stop, or significant blows to the head. See treatment of cervical spine injuries, page 90.

Buck Tilton and Frank Hubbell, in their excellent book *Medicine for the Backcountry* (The Globe Pequot Press), state, "Do not let fear of spinal cord injury blind you to more immediate threats to life. If the scene is not safe, the patient may need to be carefully moved. If the airway is not open, grasp the sides of your patient's head firmly, and pull with steady, gentle traction and attempt to align the head and neck with the rest of the body. Gentle traction should be maintained until mechanical stabilization can be improvised." (See spinal cord management on page 131.)

Focused Survey

The Physical Exam

While the purpose of the initial survey (formerly called the primary or hasty survey) is to rapidly find and correct life-threatening conditions, the focused survey (formerly identified as the secondary survey) is an attempt to identify all of the medical problems that the patient might have. This requires a thorough examination because sometimes an obvious injury can be distracting. A broken bone may cause both you and the victim to not notice a less painful but potentially more serious injury elsewhere.

The only way to perform a focused survey is to do it thoroughly, using both your vision and sense of touch, asking simple questions, and being methodical in the approach. Sense of touch is important. Sliding your hand under the victim might find areas of tenderness, even considerable blood loss that would otherwise be unnoticed. It is surprising how much blood can be absorbed into snow or sand under a wounded victim and not even noticed until your hand encounters it.

The mission of the focused survey is not only to discover various medical problems, but also to record and keep track of them during periodic reassessments. The reassessment information is even more important than the first set of information taken during the initial focused survey. How often the secondary survey needs to be repeated and how extensive it needs to be depends primarily on the history of the event. Very serious appearing events could initially require total body reassessment every 15 minutes. There can be no hard and fast rule concerning how often to repeat and how extensive the reassessments must be. There is no escaping the use of common sense. Eventually reassessment every few hours, even discontinuing this process, will become proper. This is particularly appropriate when the examination is unchanged, stable, the patient is alert, and you have obviously effectively dealt with the injuries. The scheme for recording this information is in the form of a SOAP note (which stands for **S**ubjective, **O**bjective, **A**ssessment, and **P**lan). An *accident form* to help you remember these concepts and information that needs to be sent to rescuers or remembered after an accident is located on page 212.

The most significant difference of wilderness first aid from the standard urban first aid is that the focused survey must also lead to treatment protocols. This methodical examination should generally start at the head and work its way to the feet. The exception could be children, where you might want to alleviate their apprehension by starting with the legs before their head. Generally starting at the head is best. Some ethnic groups demand this. For example, gypsies find it insulting to be touched above the waist directly after being touched below the waist. This is good to know if you are camping with gypsies.

General Principles of the Focused Survey

1. Start at the top and work your way down.
2. Move the patient as little as possible and try not to aggravate known injuries while looking for others.
3. Constantly communicate with the patient during the examination, even if she seems unconscious.
4. Look for damage, even cutting away clothing if necessary to visualize suspected injuries.
5. Ask about pain, discomfort, and abnormal sensations constantly during the exam.
6. Gently feel all relevant body parts for abnormalities.

Vital Signs

While even accurate measurements of the body's functions do not indicate what is wrong with a patient, the second and subsequent measurements indicate how well the patient is doing. You will need to use common sense to determine how often the signs are taken, but certainly close monitoring of the patient should be continued until she is "out of the woods," either literally or figuratively.

Vital signs consist of several elements: level of consciousness, pulse, respirations, skin signs, and blood pressure.

Level of Consciousness

Is the patient alert, or does she respond only to verbal or painful stimulus? Or is she unresponsive? She should know who she is, where she is, what happened to her, and about what time of the day it is. Consciousness ranges from ALERT, to VERBAL (responsive to spoken contact), PAIN (not responsive to verbal contact but responsive to being pinched or rubbed on the shin), to UNRESPONSIVE.

Pulse

Check and record rate, rhythm, and quality (thready, normal, or bounding). If an injury has been sustained by a limb, check pulses on both injured and uninjured limbs and compare.

See shock, page 16.

Deformed fracture causing a decreased pulse, see page 126.

Respirations

Note the rate, rhythm, and quality (labored, with pain, flaring of nostrils, or noise such as snores, squeaks, gurgles, or gasps). An adult normally breathes twelve to eighteen times per minute, while children breathe faster.

Respiratory difficulties, see page 17.

Skin

Check skin color and note whether it is hot/cold and moist/dry.

Hot, fever, see page 28 and *hyperthermia,* see page 202.

Cold, shock, see page 16 and *hypothermia,* see page 194.

Yellow skin, jaundice, see page 178 and *anemia,* see page 30.

Blood Pressure

Blood pressure can be measured with a stethoscope and blood pressure cuff or by estimating. If you can feel a pulse in the radial artery at the wrist, the BP top (systolic) pressure is probably at least 80 mm. If you can only feel the femoral pulse in the groin, the pressure is no lower than 70 mm. When only the carotid pulse in the neck is palpable, the systolic is probably at least 60 mm. Normal systolic blood pressures range from 100 to 140. Low upper blood pressures with normal pulses (say the 70 to 85 beats per minute range) are safe. But an increased pulse rate with a low pressure is an indication of shock.

Medical History and Physical Examination

Taking a medical history allows you to factor in your patients' previous or current illnesses as they may relate to the situation at hand. Before or during your actual physical examination, if the patients are not in an acute stage, ask about any allergies, medications that your patients are taking, past history of their health, last food or drink, and about the events that led up to the accident. If they are in pain, ask what provokes it, does it radiate, how severe is it, what type is it (burning, sharp, dull), and what time did it start?

Head

Look for damage, discoloration, and blood or fluid draining from ears, nose, and mouth. Ask about loss of consciousness, pain, or any abnormal sensations. Feel for lumps or other deformities.

Losses of consciousness, see page 13
Headache, see page 34
Ear trauma, see page 53
Eye trauma, see pages 41, 45
Nose trauma, see page 48
Mouth trauma, see page 55

Neck

Look for obvious damage, or deviation of the windpipe (trachea). Ask about pain and discomfort. Feel along the cervical spine for a pain response.

Cervical spine trauma, see page 129

Chest

Compress the ribs from both sides, as if squeezing a birdcage, keeping your hands wide to prevent the possibility of too much direct pressure on fractures. Look for damage or deformities. Ask about pain. Feel for instability.

> *Chest trauma,* see page 151.
> *Difficulty breathing,* see page 17.

Abdomen

With hands spread wide, press gently on the abdomen. Look for damage. Ask about pain and discomfort. Feel for rigidity, distention, or muscle spasms.

> *Abdominal pain,* see page 64

Back

Slide your hands under the patient, palpating as much of the spine as possible.

> *Spine trauma,* see page 131

Pelvis/Hip

Place your hands on the top front of the pelvis on both sides (the iliac crests), pressing gently down, and pulling toward the midline of the body. Ask about pain. Feel for instability.

> *Hip or pelvis pain,* see page 145.

Legs

With your hands surrounding each leg, one at a time, run from the groin down to the toes, squeezing as you go. Note especially if there is a lack of circulation, sensation, or motion in the toes.

> *Bone injury,* see fractures on page 125.

Shoulders and Arms

One at a time, with hands wide, squeeze each shoulder, and run down the arms to the fingers. Check for circulation, sensation, and motion in the fingers.

> *Shoulder trauma,* see page 133.
> *Joint trauma,* see page 124.
> *Broken bone,* see page 125.
> *Bruises,* see page 136.

Shock

Shock is a deficiency in oxygen supply reaching the brain and other tissues as a result of decreased circulation. An important aspect of the correction of shock is to identify and treat the underlying cause. Shock can be caused by burns, electrocution, hypothermia, bites, stings, bleeding, fractures, pain, hyperthermia, high altitude cerebral edema, illness, rough handling, allergic reaction (anaphylaxis), damage or excitement to the central nervous system, dehydration from sweating, vomiting or diarrhea, or loss of adequate heart strength. Each of these underlying causes is discussed separately in this text.

Shock can progress through several stages before death results. The first phase is called the "compensatory stage" during which the body attempts to counter the damage by increasing its activity level. Arteries constrict and the pulse rate increases, thus maintaining the blood pressure. The next phase is called the "progressive stage," when suddenly the blood pressure drops and the patient becomes worse, often swiftly. When he has reached the "irreversible stage," vital organs have suffered from loss of oxygen so profoundly that death occurs even with aggressive treatment.

Consider the possibility of shock in any victim of an accident or when significant illness develops. Ensure that an adequate airway is established (see further discussion under Rescue Breathing, page 19). Assess the cardiovascular status. Place your hand over the carotid artery (Figure 1.1) to obtain the pulse. In compensatory shock the patient will have a weak, rapid pulse. In adults the rate will be over 140, in children 180 beats per minute. If there is doubt about a pulse being present, listen to the bare chest. If cardiac standstill is present, begin one-person or two-person CPR (see pages 19–22). Elevate the legs to 45° to obtain a better return of venous blood to the heart and head. However, if there has been a severe head injury, keep the person flat. If he has trouble breathing, elevate the chest and head to a comfortable position. Protect the patient from the environment with insulation under and shelter up above. Strive to make him comfortable. Watch your spoken and body language. Reassure without patronizing and let nothing that you say or act out cause him increased distress.

Attempt to treat the underlying cause of the shock. The primary or secondary survey and history may well elicit the cause of shock and appropriate treatment can be devised from the field-expedient methods listed in this book.

Decision/Care Table

Shock due to severe allergic reactions is called "anaphylactic shock" and is discussed on page 154.

Difficult Respirations

It has been stated that you can live three minutes without air, three days without water, three weeks without food, and three months without love. Some feel that these categories might stretch their time limits to four, others would feel shorter periods might be lethal. Without any question, adequate respirations are the most significant demand of the living creature. When respiratory difficulties start, it's urgent to find the reason and alleviate it. When they stop, reestablishing the air flow is critical.

Foreign Body Airway Obstruction

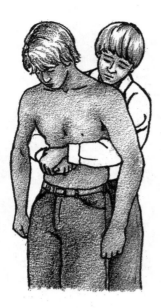

If a conscious adult seems to be having distressed breathing, ask "Are you choking?" If they apparently are, perform an abdominal thrust or the Heimlich Maneuver, to relieve foreign-body airway obstruction or choking. If the victim is standing or sitting, stand behind and wrap your arms around the patient, proceeding as follows: Make a fist with one hand. Place the thumb side of the fist against the victim's abdomen, in the midline slightly above the navel and well below the breastbone. Grasp your fist with the other hand. Press the fist into the victim's abdomen with a quick, upward thrust. Each new thrust should be a separate and distinct movement. It may be necessary to repeat the thrust multiple times to clear the airway. If the person is obese or pregnant, use chest thrusts in the same manner as just described, but with the hands around the lower chest.

Figure 1-2: The Heimlich Maneuver

If the victim becomes unconscious and is on the ground, the victim should be placed on her back, face up. In civilization activate the EMS system. Perform a tongue–jaw lift, followed by a finger sweep to remove the object. Open the airway and try to ventilate. If still obstructed, reposition the head and try to ventilate again. Give up to five abdominal thrusts, then repeat the tongue–jaw lift, finger sweep, and attempt ventilation. Repeat these steps until effective.

To perform an abdominal thrust with the patient on the ground, the rescuer kneels astride the victim's thighs. The rescuer places the heel of one hand against the victim's abdomen, in the midline slightly above the navel and well below the breastbone, and the second hand directly on top of the first. The rescuer then presses into the abdomen with quick upward thrusts.

Adult One-Rescuer Cardiopulmonary Resuscitation (CPR)

To establish unresponsiveness, first try talking—clearly and loudly—to the victim and ask questions such as "Are you OK? Can you hear me?" If there is no response to your verbal contact, make gentle physical contact by touching the victim's shoulder and repeating your questions. In civilization activate the Emergency Medical Response system prior to attempting CPR. In the wilderness immediately proceed with the following steps.

Open the airway using the head-tilt/chin-lift or jaw-thrust technique (see Figure 1–3). Place one hand on the victim's forehead and apply firm, backward pressure with the palm to tilt the head back. Also place the fingers of the other hand under the bony part of the lower jaw near the chin and lift to bring the chin forward and the teeth almost shut, thus supporting the jaw and helping to tilt the head back, as indicated in Figure 1–3. In case of suspected neck injury, use the chin-lift without the head-tilt technique. The nose is pinched shut by using the thumb and index finger of the hand on the forehead.

The chin-lift method will place tension on the tongue and throat structures to ensure that the air passage will open. This opening of the air passage may be all that is required to allow the victim to start breathing again. Reassess breathing again by looking for the chest rising or falling, listening for air escaping during expiration, and feeling the movement of air.

If breathing is absent, give 2 slow breaths (1½ to 2 seconds per

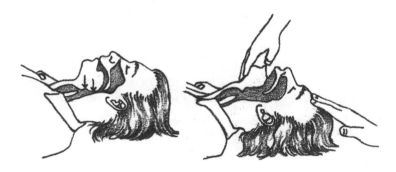

Figure 1-3: The head-tilt/chin-lift method of opening the airway in an unconscious person. ©*Banyan International Corp., used by permission.*

breath), watching the chest rise. Then allow for exhalation between breaths. The breathing rate should be once every 5 to 6 seconds, about 12 breaths per minute. Using slow, full breaths reduces the amount of air that tends to enter the stomach and cause gastric distention.

Check the carotid pulse. This is found by placing your hand on the voicebox (larynx). Slip the tips of your fingers into the groove beside the voicebox and feel for the pulse (see Figure 1–1). If breathing is absent but pulse is present, provide rescue breathing at the rate of about 12 breaths per minute. If there is no pulse, give cycles of 15 chest compressions (at a rate of 80 to 100 compressions per minute), followed by 2 slow breaths.

Chest compressions are performed by the rescuer kneeling at the victim's side, near his chest, locating the notch at the lowest portion of his breastbone (sternum). Place the heel of one hand on the sternum 1½ to 2 inches above this notch. Place the other hand on top of the one that is in position on the sternum. See Figure 1–4. Be sure to keep your fingers off the ribs. The easiest way to prevent this is to interlock your fingers, thus keeping them confined to the sternum. With your shoulders directly over the victim's sternum, compress downward keeping your arms straight. Depress the sternum 1½ to 2 inches for an average adult victim. Relax the pressure completely, keeping your hands in contact with the sternum at all times, but allowing the sternum to return to its normal position between compressions. Both compression and relaxation should be of equal duration.

Perform 15 external chest compressions at a rate of 80 to 100 per minute. Open the airway and deliver 2 rescue breaths. Locate the proper hand position and begin 15 more compressions at a rate of 80 to 100 per minute, then 2 slow breaths. Perform 4 complete cycles of 15 compressions followed by 2 slow breaths.

After 4 cycles of 15:2 compressions and ventilations (about 1 minute), reevaluate the patient. Check for the return of the carotid pulse (5 seconds). If it is absent, resume CPR with 15 compressions followed by 2 slow breaths, as indicated above. If it is present, continue to the next step.

Check breathing (3 to 5 seconds). If present, monitor breathing and pulse closely. If absent, perform rescue breathing at 12 times per minute and monitor pulse closely.

If CPR is continued, stop and check for return of pulse and spontaneous breathing after each 4 cycles. Do not interrupt CPR for more than 5 seconds except in special circumstances.

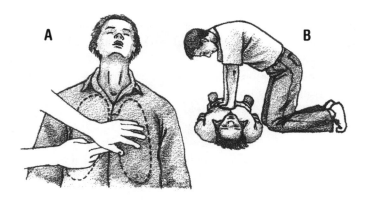

A

B

Figure 1-4: A. Position of hands. B. Position of rescuer.

Once CPR is started it should be maintained until professional assistance can take over the responsibility, or until a physician declares the patient dead. If CPR has been continued for 30 minutes without regaining cardiac function, and the eyes are fixed and non-reactive to light, the patient can be presumed dead. The exceptions would be hypothermia (see page 194) and lightning injuries (page 204). In these circumstances, if professional help does not intervene, CPR should be continued until the rescuers are exhausted.

Some authorities in wilderness rescue have felt that the survival rate is so low without defibrillation within 4 minutes by paramedics, that CPR should not be started in the bush when cardiac standstill is due to a heart attack. It certainly should not be started or maintained under these conditions when its performance might endanger the lives of members of the rescue party. Regardless, learning CPR is an important skill that every person should master. *The only way to learn this technique is to take a CPR course—it cannot be properly self-taught.*

Adult Two-Rescuer CPR

The two-rescuer technique differs in that Rescuer One will take a position by the head and Rescuer Two assumes the position as described under one-rescuer CPR. While breathing and compression rates are the same, the ratios are different.

After establishing unresponsiveness (and activating the EMS system if in civilization), Rescuer One opens the airway (head-tilt/chin-lift or jaw thrust) and checks for breathing (look, feel, listen). Rescuer One then gives 2 slow breaths (1½ to 2 seconds per breath), watches the chest rise, and allows for exhalation between breaths. After the 2 breaths, Rescuer One checks the carotid pulse.

If there is no pulse, Rescuer Two gives cycles of 5 chest compressions (rate of 80 to 100 compressions per minute), followed by 1 slow breath by Rescuer One. After 1 minute of rescue support, Rescuer One again checks the pulse. If there is no pulse, this 5:1 compression:breathing cycle is continued, with reassessment after each minute.

Two person CPR is not generally taught to the public in basic courses to avoid confusion with the ratios and rates of the compressions and respirations of one person CPR. However, in the wilderness where prolonged CPR might be necessary, being familiar with this technique can help alleviate the tremendous fatigue that CPR induces in rescuers.

Rapid Breathing

Rapid breathing (*hyperventilation syndrome* or *tachypnea*) can represent either a serious medical condition or can be the result of a harmless panic attack. This symptom in a diabetic is very dangerous, but can be prevented by proper diabetic management. High altitude stress can result in hyperventilation (see page 207). See the Table on page 17 for additional diagnosis of a rapid or difficult breathing disorder.

The feeling of panic that results in very shallow breathing causes the victim to lose excessive amounts of carbon dioxide from the bloodstream. The resulting change in the acid–base balance of the blood (respiratory alkalosis) will cause a numb feeling around the mouth, in the extremities, and if the breathing pattern persists, it can even lead to violent spasms of the hands and feet. This is a form of hysteria that can appear in teenagers and healthy young adults. It would be helpful for victims to rebreathe their air from a stuff sack to increase the carbon dioxide level in their bloodstream. They need to be reassured and told to slow down the breathing. It is fine for them to draw long, deep breaths as it is the rapid breathing that causes the loss of so much carbon dioxide.

If necessary, from the Non-Rx Oral Medication Module give Percogesic 2 tablets or from the Rx Oral/Topical Medication Module give

Atarax 25mg, 2 tablets. The Rx Injectable Medication Module Vistaril 50 mg IM is also helpful in treating hyperventilation. These drugs are being used in this instance as antianxiety drugs.

Cardiac Evaluation and Care

Heart Attack—Myocardial Infarction

The following symptoms are fairly classic for a person having an inadequate oxygen supply to the heart: chest heaviness or pain with exertion; pain or ache radiating into the neck or into the arms; sweating, clammy, pale appearance; shortness of breath. The pain is called *angina* and results from the heart muscle starving for oxygen. If the blockage is profound, heart muscle will die. This is called a *myocardial infarction* and it means heart attack and damaged muscle. The cause of death is frequently a profound irregular heartbeat caused by electrical irritation in the damaged muscle. Another cause of death is loss of adequate power to pump blood from weakened heart muscle. A delayed cause of death can be from the sudden rupture of the weakened heart wall.

The most important thing for an individual in the wilderness with these symptoms is rest. Rest causes the oxygen requirement of the heart to be at a minimum. Position the victim for optimum comfort, generally with his head elevated about 45 degrees, see Figure 1–5. In some cases, even with an electrocardiogram, it is impossible for a trained physician to determine whether or not an individual is having a cardiac problem. When in doubt—rest the patient and try to evacuate without having him do any of the work. Treat as a total invalid.

Give the patient one regular size aspirin (324 mg) or two baby aspirin (81 mg each) immediately. Check to see if the victim is carrying any prescription heart medications and note usage instructions on the bottle. Give sublingual nitroglycerine if anyone in the party is carrying it. One tablet, followed by two more at 5 minute intervals would be appropriate. You may give the victim medication adequate to relieve pain (see page 30). From the Rx Oral Module give Atarax (hydroxyzine) 25 mg orally, or from the Rx Injectable Module Vistaril (hydroxyzine) 25 mg IM, if needed to treat nausea or to help sedate the victim. You may repeat the pain medication and the nausea/sedation medication every 4 hours as needed.

Observe respirations and pulse rate. You will note the comment in the

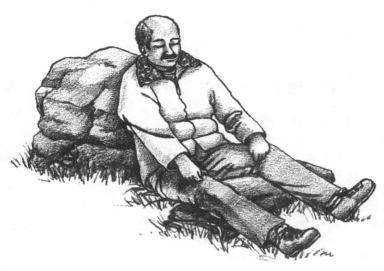

Figure 1-5: A heart attack victim can usually breathe better sitting up.

section under Adult-One Rescuer CPR that providing CPR to a heart attack victim who cannot be defibrillated within four minutes is a lost cause. The only significant reason for starting CPR, if the person becomes pulseless, is to placate the onlookers. Due to the virtual zero salvage rate, you are treating yourself and the others watching who, after perhaps half an hour, will consider that everything has been done that was possible. This may be a very important part of the emotional support required by individual group members as they reflect back upon the event.

Rapid Heart Rate

Tachycardia

A rapid heart rate after trauma or other stress may signify impending shock. The underlying cause should be treated. This may require fluid replacement or pain medication. Body temperature elevations cause an increase in heart rate of ten beats per minute for each degree above normal. At elevations above 8,000 feet (2,500 meters), a pulse rate of 120 or greater per minute after a twenty minute rest is an early sign of pulmonary edema (see page 208). A sudden onset of rapid heart rate with sharp chest pain can indicate a pulmonary embolism or pneumothorax. Treat with pain medication and have the patient sit propped up for ease in breathing.

A very rapid rate of 140 to 220 beats per minute may be encountered suddenly and without warning in very healthy individuals. This PAT (paroxysmal atrial tachycardia) frequently has as its first symptom, a feeling of profound weakness. The victim generally stops what she is doing and feels better sitting down. These attacks are self-limited, but they can be aborted by one of several maneuvers that stimulate the vagus nerve, which in turn slows down the pulse rate. These maneuvers include: holding one's breath and bearing down very hard; closing one's eyes and pressing firmly on the eyeballs; inducing vomiting with a finger down the throat; or feeling for the carotid pulse in the neck and gently pressing on the enlarged portion of this vessel, one side at a time. Another effective maneuver is to take a deep breath and plunge one's face into ice water. Frequently, however, the victim must just wait for the attack to pass. This arrhythmia will sometimes come on after a spate of activity. No medication is generally required.

Slow Heart Rate

Bradycardia

A slow heart rate is important in two instances: when someone passes out and when it accompanies a high fever. Generally fainting or shock is associated with a rapid pulse rate (see compensatory shock, page 16), an attempt by the body to maintain blood pressure. A safety mechanism, which the body employs to prevent blood pressure from elevating too high, is a sensor system in each carotid artery in the neck, called the carotid bodies. If these sensors are stimulated by an elevated blood pressure, a reflex mechanism that relaxes and opens blood vessels throughout the body and lowers the heart rate is generated via impulses from the carotid bodies through the vagus nerve. The vagus nerve can be fooled into inappropriately initiating this reflex mechanism at times. A person watching an accident scene, or even thinking about such an episode, can stimulate the vagus nerve through its connection with the frontal lobe. The resulting slow pulse and relaxed arteries can result in the person passing out.

As mentioned above, the pulse usually increases as the body temperature rises. It also falls as the core temperature lowers into a hypothermia state (see page 194). Several diseases are notable in that the pulse rate is lower than would be expected for the elevated body temperature caused by the disease. Typhoid fever (page 190) is the classic example of this phenomena.

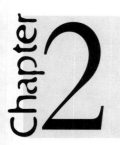

Chapter 2

Body System Symptoms and Management

Symptom Management

Symptoms are indicators of problems. Fever, pain, and itch can sometimes aid you in determining exactly what is wrong with the patient. The various decision tables in this book use one or more symptoms to help identify a diagnosis and plan a treatment.

It is also useful to know how to minimize some of these symptoms. Why itch when you can treat it? The cause of an itch may vary from poison plant dermatitis to an insect bite to liver disease. Regardless of the cause, what can you do to alleviate it?

The best method for reducing symptoms is to successfully treat the underlying problem. Sometimes definitive treatment cannot be accomplished. At other times, the symptom remains after the injury is past and the symptom becomes the greatest part of the problem.

Table 2–1 provides a guide to general symptom care.

General Symptom Care Guide	Table 2-1

For a discussion of symptoms localized to a particular body part, refer to Table 2–2 for the anatomical or body location and symptom cross-referenced in the Clinical Reference Index, starting on page 238.

Table 2-2 General Anatomical Location Guide

Eye	35
Nose	47
Ear	49
Mouth (and dental)	55
Chest	62
Abdomen	64
Genitalia	74

Evaluation and management of symptoms relating to injuries and environmental exposure can also be found through the Clinical Reference Index.

Fever/Chills

The average oral temperature of a resting individual is 98.6° F (37° C); in active individuals it is 101° F (38° C). Rectal temperatures are 0.5 to 1° Fahrenheit higher. A temperature rise in a human will result in the heart rate increasing ten beats per minute faster than the patient's normal resting temperature. This is a useful field method of judging temperature, if each individual knows what his resting pulse is. Some diseases cause a peculiar drop in heart rate, even in the face of an obviously high temperature. The most notable of these are typhoid fever, page 190 and yellow fever, page 192.

Although injury and exposure can cause elevated body temperature, fever is usually the result of infection. The cause of the fever should be sought and treated. If pain or infection is located in the ear, throat, etc., refer to the appropriate anatomical area listed in the Clinical Reference Index at the end of the book.

If other symptoms beside fever are present (diarrhea, cough, etc.), see the cross–references listing these symptoms in the Clinical Reference Index in order to provide treatment to alleviate the suffering of these conditions. This may diagnose the underlying disease, which will have a specific treatment indicated in the text.

The wilderness approach to therapy may be quite different from that used in clinical medicine. In the wilderness, when in doubt about whether or not the fever is due to viral, bacterial, or other infectious causes, treat for a bacterial infection with antibiotic from your Rx medication modules. Initially, give the patient Levaquin 500 mg, 1 tablet daily and continue until the fever has broken for an additional 3 days. This will conserve medication while providing adequate antibiotic coverage to a suspected bacterial infection. If it is possible that the patient has a strep throat, give Zithromax rather than Levaquin, as described on page 55. If you are not carrying the Rx kit, then treat the symptoms using the medications described in your non-Rx kits. In either case, rest is important until the patient is again free of fever and has a sense of well being.

Chills are a kind of shivering, accompanied by a feeling of coldness (not related to hypothermia, see page 194). Chills are usually followed by fever. They frequently indicate the onset of a bacterial infection, which should be treated with an antibiotic as described above.

People tolerate fevers quite well and it is possible that elevated temperatures enhance the immune response to infections. However, persons with a history of febrile seizures or a history of heart problems should certainly be treated to lower an elevated temperature. Generally it is best to use Tylenol (acetaminophen), but usually ibuprofen and aspirin are safe. Aspirin should be avoided in children with chicken pox or other viral illness due to an increase in Reye's syndrome with its use (a disease of progressive liver failure and brain deterioration). The non-Rx Oral Medication Module contains two products useful in treating fever, ibuprofen and Percogesic. As these are over the counter products, the dosage will be listed on the product containers.

Lethargy

Lethargy, or prolonged tiredness or malaise, is a non–localizing symptom such as fever or muscle ache (myalgia). Pain, however, is a localizing symptom that points to the organ system that may be the cause of such things as lethargy, fever, or a generally ill feeling. Frequently after a few days of lethargy—or at times even hours—localizing symptoms develop and the cause of the lethargy can be determined to be an infection of the throat, ear, etc.

Sometimes a chronic condition is the source of the lethargy, such as anemia, leukemia, low thyroid function, depression, occult or low-grade infection, mental depression, or even physical exhaustion. The latter we would expect to be obvious from the history of the preceding level of activity and strength should return within a few days.

Anemia can be present due to chronic blood loss from ulcers, menstrual problems, inadequate formation of iron, leukemia, or other cancers in the bone marrow, etc. Chronic anemia can be identified by looking at the color of the skin inside the lower eye lids. Pull the lower lid down and look at it. Compare to another person. Normally this thin skin is very orange colored, even if the cheeks are pale. If the color is a blanched white, anemia is very likely. Another good indication of anemia is an increase in the pulse rate of more than 30 beats per minute in the standing position, compared to a recumbent position.

Malaise or lethargy can be a presenting complaint of acute mountain sickness, but this would be unusual below 6,000 feet. If other symptoms are present such as nausea, one must think of hepatitis (see page 178), or if preceded by a severe sore throat, infectious mononucleosis (see page 55). Lethargy is one of the most common presenting complaints that I see in my office. An accurate diagnosis requires careful evaluation, sometimes aided by laboratory tests. If the problem is not depression, then regardless of the cause, the person needs rest, proper nutrition, and adequate shelter.

Pain

Adequate pain management can involve a mixture of proper medication and attitude—the attitudes of both the victim and the medic are crucial. A calm, professional approach to problems will lessen anxiety, panic, and pain. Pain is an important symptom that tells you something is wrong. It generally "localizes" or points to the exact cause of the trouble, so that pain in various parts of the body will be your clue that a problem exists and that specific treatment may be required to eliminate it. Refer to the Clinical Reference Index (page 238) under specific areas of the body (such as ear, abdomen, etc.) to read about diagnosis and specific treatments of the causes of pain.

An application of cold water or ice can frequently relieve pain. This is very important in burns, orthopedic injuries, and skin irritations. Cold can sometimes relieve muscle spasm. Gentle massage and local hot compresses are also effective treatments for muscle spasm.

The alleviation of pain with medication calls for a step-wise increase in medication strength until relief is obtained. Throughout this book you will be referred to this section for adequate pain management. Use discretion in providing adequate medication to do the job, without overdosing the patient. Remember that a pill takes about 20 minutes to begin working and is at maximum therapeutic strength in about 1 hour. If possible, wait an hour to see how effective the medication has been. But use common sense. If the injury is severe, give a respectable initial dose.

Mild Pain

For mild pain, from the Non-Rx Oral Medication Module provide the victim with Percogesic, 1 or 2 tablets every 4 hours. Percogesic is probably the best pain medication that can be obtained without a prescription, providing both pain and muscle relaxant actions. It is fully described on page 220. It is particularly good for orthopedic injuries or whenever muscle sprains and contusions are encountered. It is also ideal for menstrual cramps, tension headache, and it is relatively safe to use in head injuries. It can also be used for the muscle aches and fever from viral and bacterial infections.

Another pain medication suggested in the Non-Rx Oral Medication Module is ibuprofen. Its anti-inflammatory abilities make it ideal for treatment of tendinitis, bursitis, or arthritic pain. Brand names generally available are Nuprin, Medipren, and Advil. An alternate selection for this product would be either a buffered aspirin or enteric-coated aspirin product.

Severe Pain

For severe pain you may have to rely on the Rx Oral/Topical Medication Module component Lorcet 10/650, taking 1 tablet every 4 to 6 hours. One of these tablets is generally enough to eliminate a bad toothache in a large adult. The total 24-hour dose should not exceed 6 tablets. They can be augmented by also giving the victim 1 or 2 Atarax 25 mg tablets every 4 to 6 hours. This medication helps eliminate the nausea associated with high hydrocodone dosages and from my experience it also potentiates the pain medication so that it works more effectively.

The Rx Oral/Topical Medication Module also contains nasally inhaled Stadol (butorphanol tartrate). This very powerful pain medication is about ten times stronger per milligram dose than morphine. It is taken as spray up one nostril, followed by another spray in the other nostril 5 to 20 minutes later, if necessary. This may be repeated every 3 to 4 hours. This medication is as powerful as any injectable product available. See full discussion of this medication on page 225. Its rate of onset is fairly rapid. Within 5 minutes relief should start, reaching its maximum effect within 20 minutes. As there are no needles required to administer this drug, it should be easier to take on foreign trips than the injectable medications. You might consider keeping it with your toothpaste until across the border. At least I do.

If you are carrying the Rx Injectable Medication Module, severe pain can be treated with an injection of 10 mg of Nubain (nalbuphine). This amounts to ½ ml of the strength listed in the kit. This can be potentiated with Vistaril (hydroxyzine) 25 mg or 50 mg, also by injection. Vistaril and Nubain can be mixed in the same syringe. They both sting upon injection.

Local pain can be eliminated or eased with cold compresses or ice as mentioned above. Applying dibucaine 1 percent ointment will help skin surface pain, such as from sunburn, abrasions, etc. Applying a cover of Spenco 2nd Skin dressing (both products are recommended for the Topical Bandaging Module) provides cooling relief due to the evaporative action of the water from this safe to use gel pad. Deep cuts and painful puncture wounds can be injected with lidocaine 1% from the Rx Injectable Medication Module. This technique is described on page 100.

Itch

As itch is a sensation that is transmitted by pain fibers, all pain medications can be used in alleviating itch sensations. Itch also indicates that something is awry and may require specific treatment. The most common causes are local allergic reactions, such as *poisonous plants, fungal infections,* and *insect bites or infestations* (or look under specific causes in the index). General principles of treatment include further avoidance of the offending substance (not so easy in the case of mosquitos). Avoid applying heat to an itchy area, as this makes it flare up worse. Avoid scratching or rubbing, this also increases the reaction. If weeping blisters have formed, apply wet soaks with a clean cloth or gauze. While plain water soaks will help, making a solution of boric acid, Epsom salts, or even regular table salt will help dry the lesions and alleviate some of the itch. Make an approximately 10% solution weight to volume of water.

Cream-based preparations work well on moist lesions, while ointments are more effective on dry, scaly ones. The Topical Bandaging Module contains 1% hydrocortisone cream, which, while safe to use, is generally not very effective against severe allergic dermatitis. For best results, one should apply it four times daily and then cover the area with an occlusive dressing, such as cellophane or a piece of polybag. The Rx

Oral/Topical Medication Module contains Topicort (desoximetasone) .25% cream, which is strong enough to adequately treat allergic dermatitis with light coats applied twice daily. Athlete's foot and skin rashes in the groin or in skin folds are generally fungal and should not be treated with these creams. They may seem to provide temporary relief, but they can actually worsen fungal infections. For possible fungal infections, apply the clotrimazole cream 1% twice daily from the Topical Bandaging Module.

Oral medications are frequently required to treat severe skin reactions and itch. The Non-Rx Oral Medication Module contains Benadryl (diphenhydramine) 25 mg. Take 1 or 2 capsules every 6 hours. It is one of the most effective antihistamines made. The Rx Oral Topical Medication Module contains Atarax (hydroxyzine) 25 mg. It is very effective in treating the symptom of itch and as an antihistamine. Take 1 or 2 tablets every 6 hours. These medications are safe to use on all sorts of itch problems. If one is suffering from an asthma attack they should not be used, however, as they tend to dry out the lung secretions and potentially make the illness worse.

Hives

Hives are the result of a severe allergic reaction. Commonly called welts, these raised red blotches develop rapidly and frequently have a red border around a clearer skin area in the center, sometimes referred to as an "annular" lesion. As these can and do appear over large surfaces of the skin, treatment with a cream is of little help. Use the diphenhydramine or hydroxyzine as indicated above. Extensive urticaria or allergic dermatitis lesion frequently need to be treated with an oral steroid. The Rx Oral/Topical Medication Module has Decadron (dexamethasone) 4 mg tablets, which should be taken 1 tablet twice daily after meals.

It should be noted that the Vistaril recommended for the Rx Injectable Module is also hydroxyzine as is the oral Atarax. This same module also has an injectable form of the dexamethasone. For treatment of rash, the oral medications should suffice.

In case of a concurrent asthmatic condition or the development of shock, treat as for *anaphylactic shock*, page 154. In case of suspected tick bite, an annular or circular lesion may be a sign of Lyme disease (see page 180). If fever is present, one must consider that a rash and itch have resulted from an infection. A diagnosis may be impossible in the bush so that treatment with antibiotic is appropriate. Use doxycycline 100 mg twice daily from the Rx Oral/Topical Medication Module as a field-expedient solution to the problem. Treat fever as described in that section on page 28.

Hiccups

Hiccups can be started by a variety of causes and are generally self-limited. Persistent hiccups can be a medically important symptom requiring professional evaluation and help in control. Several approaches to their control in camp may be tried. Have the victim hold his breath for as long as possible or re-breathe air from a stuff sack. These maneuvers raise the carbon dioxide level and help stop the hiccup reflex mechanism. Drinking 5 to 6 ounces of ice water fast sometimes works; one may also close one's eyes and press firmly on the eyeballs to stimulate the vagal blockage of the hiccup. The other vagus nerve stimulation maneuvers indicated under PAT, page 25, can be tried.

If these maneuvers do not work, from the Non-Rx Oral Medication Module give Percogesic 2 tablets or from the Rx Oral/Topical Medication Module you may give Atarax 25 mg, 2 tablets. In the Rx Injectable Medication Module Vistaril is an injectable form of Atarax. This medication may be given in a dose of 50 mg IM. These doses may be repeated every 4 hours. Let the patient rest and try to avoid bothering him until bedtime. If still symptomatic at that point, have him re-breathe the air from inside his sleeping bag, to raise the carbon dioxide level in his bloodstream and, if nothing else, to muffle the sounds.

Headache

A variety of problems can cause a headache; refer to Table 2–3. Too much sun exposure, dehydration, withdrawal from caffeine, stress, high altitude illness, dental or eye problems—the list is almost endless. Be sure to consider the possible underlying problems mentioned above as they are the most common.

Table 2-3

Causes of Headache Guide

Dental	59
TMJ	54
High altitude	207
Heat	202
Sun exposure	41

Eye

Pain and irritation of the eye can be devastating. Causes that might be encountered in a remote-area trip are listed in Table 2–4.

Symptoms and Signs of Eye Pathology						Table 2-4
	Vision Loss	Pain	Red	Drainage	Tissue Swelling	
Trauma (39)	●	■	■	●	●	
Foreign Body (36)	■	■	■			
Infection:						
bacteria (43)	●	■		■	●	
viral (42)	●	■	●	●		
sty (44)	●	■		■		
Allergy (44)	■	●				
Corneal Ulcers (36, 39)	●			■		
Snow Blindness (41)	●		■	■	●	
Strain		●				
Glaucoma (46)		●		■		
Spontaneous Subconjunctival (45) Hemorrhage (45)	■					

Legend:
■ A frequent or intense symptom
● Common, less intense symptom
Blank Less likely to produce this symptom

Note: The page numbers are in brackets.

Eye Patch and Bandaging Techniques

In case of evidence of infection, do not use an eye patch or splint, but have the patient wear dark glasses, a wide-brimmed hat, or take other measures to decrease light exposure. Wash the eye with clean water by dabbing with wet, clean cloth every two hours to remove pus and excess secretions. Apply antibiotics as indicated under *eye infections.*

Eye patch techniques must allow for gentle closure of the eyelid and retard blinking activity. Sometimes both eyes must be patched for this to succeed, but this obviously is a hardship for the patient. Simple strips of tape holding the eyelids shut may suffice. In case of trauma, an annular ring of cloth may be constructed to pad the eye without pressure over the eyeball. A simple eye patch with oversize gauze or cloth may work fine, as the bone of the orbital rim around the eye acts to protect the eyeball, which is recessed.

Serious injury requires patching both eyes, as movement in the injured eye will decrease if movement in the unaffected eye is also controlled. It generally helps to have the victim kept at rest with her head elevated 30 degrees. A severe blow to one eye may cause temporary blindness in both eyes, which can resolve in hours to days. Obviously a person with loss of vision should be treated by a physician if possible. Eye dressings must be removed, or at least changed, in 24 hours.

If a foreign object has been removed from the eye or the victim has suffered a corneal abrasion, the best splint is the tension patch. Start by placing two gauze pads over the shut eye, requesting the patient to keep his eyes closed until the bandaging is completed. The patient may help hold the gauze in place. Three pieces of one-inch-wide tape are ideal, long enough to extend from the center of the forehead to just below the cheekbone. Fasten the first piece of tape to the center of the forehead, extending the tape diagonally downward across the eye patch. The second and third strips are applied parallel to the first strip, one above and the other below. This dressing will result in firm splinting of the bandaged eye.

Foreign Body Eye Injury

The most common eye problems in the wilderness will be foreign body, abrasion, snow blindness and infection (conjunctivitis). Therapy for these problems is virtually the same, except that it is very important to remove any foreign body that may be present.

The initial step in examining the painful eye is to remove the pain. One of the lessons drilled into medical students is to never, never write a prescription for eye anesthesia agents (such as the tetracaine ophthalmic solution that I recommend for the Rx Oral/Topical Medication Module). The reason is the patient may use it, obtain relief, and then not have the eye carefully examined for a foreign body. Eventually this foreign body may cause an ulcer to form in the cornea, doing profound damage. When using the tetracaine, remember that it is very important to find and remove any foreign body. Pull down on the lower lid and use one drop. If the patient is unable to open her eye due to pain, just place one or two drops in the inner corner of the eye with her lying face up. Have her blink once or twice to allow the liquid to cover the eyeball. This medication burns when initially placed in the eye. This will increase the level of pain for a brief period until the medication takes effect. After the patient has calmed down, have her open the eye and look straight ahead. Very carefully shine a pen light at the cornea from one side to see if a minute speck becomes visible. By moving the light back and forth, one might see movement of a shadow on the iris of the eye and thus confirm the presence of a foreign body. Mucous can give a gooey appearance to the cornea that may mimic a foreign body. Have the victim blink to move any mucous around. A point that consistently stays put with blinking is probably a foreign body.

In making the foreign body examination, also be sure to check under the eyelids. Evert the upper lid over a Q-tip stick, thus examining not only the eyeball, but also the under-surface of the eyelid. This surface may be gently brushed with the cotton applicator to eliminate minute particles. Always use a fresh Q-tip when touching the eye or eyelid each additional time. Some foreign bodies can be removed easily. Have the patient place his face under water and blink. Water turbulence from under-water blinking or turbulence from directing running water from a fast moving stream or by pouring from a cup may wash the problem away.

When a foreign body has been found imbedded in the cornea, take a sterile, or at least a clean, Q-tip and approach the foreign body from the side. Gently prod it with the Q-tip handle until it is loosened. The surface of the eye will indent under the pressure of this scraping action. Indeed the surface of the cornea will be scratched in the maneuver, but it will quickly heal. Once the foreign body has been dislodged, if it does not stick to the wooden or plastic handle but slides loose along the corneal surface, use the cotton portion to touch it for removal.

A stoic individual, particularly one accustomed to contact lenses, might be able to undergo a non-complicated foreign body removal without the use of tetracaine .5% ophthalmic drops, but using anesthesia makes the patient more comfortable and cuts down on interference from the blink reflex.

Foreign bodies stuck in the cornea can be very stubborn and resist removal. At times it is necessary to pick them loose with the sharp point of a #11 scalpel blade or the tip of a needle (I frequently use an 18 gauge needle). Anesthesia with tetracaine will be a necessity for this procedure. Scraping with these instruments will cause a more significant scratch to the corneal surface, but under these circumstances it may have to be accepted. I would leave stubborn foreign bodies for removal by a physician in all but the most desperate circumstances. If you have a difficult time removing an obvious foreign body from the surface of the cornea, a wait of two to three days may allow the cornea to ulcerate slightly so that removal with the Q-tip stick may be much easier. Deeply lodged foreign bodies will have to be left for surgical removal.

A painless foreign body may not be a foreign body. It could be a rust ring left behind after a bit of ferrous, or iron-containing, material has fallen out of the eye after having been lodged for a short time. If what you see is painless, ignore it in the wilderness setting.

The history of striking an object should alert you to the fact that the injury may have penetrated much more deeply than you would expect from blowing debris hitting the eye. While blowing debris can lodge in the eye surface, a foreign body slamming into the eye due to someone striking an object (say, a hammer against a rock) might have penetrated very deeply into the eyeball. Penetrating injuries are a disaster!

A puncture wound of the eyelid mandates careful examination of the cornea surface for evidence of a penetrating foreign body. These injuries must be seen by a physician for surgical care. Evacuation is necessary. If this is impossible, the eye must be patched, examined for infection twice daily, and treated with antibiotic both by mouth and with ointment.

After removal of a foreign body, or even after scraping the eye while attempting to remove one, apply some antibiotic. The prescription kit should contain Tobradex ophthalmic drops. There are no non-prescription eye antibiotics. Brand name Neosporin and Polysporin ointments in 15 gram tubes are non-prescription antibiotics that can be used in the eye. However the manufacturer cannot recommend the use of these over-the-counter products for this purpose.

While the tetracaine will provide local pain relief, continued use may hinder the natural healing process and may disguise a significant injury or the presence of an additional foreign body. Pain relief is best attempted by patching the eye, providing a damp cloth for evaporative cooling, and oral pain medication. Percogesic or ibuprofen 200 mg from the non-Rx kit, both given in a dose of 2 tablets every 4 to 6 hours, may be provided for pain. The prescription analgesic Lorcet 10/650 1 tablet every 4 to 6 hours, would provide significant pain relief.

Contact Lenses

The increased popularity of contact lens wear means that several problems associated with their use have also increased. The lenses are of two basic types. The hard or rigid lens, which generally is smaller and does not extend beyond the iris, and the soft lens, which does extend beyond the iris onto the white of the eye. Soft lenses have been designed for extended wear. Hard lens use requires frequent removal, as the delicate cornea of the eye obtains oxygen from the environment and nutrient from eye secretions. These lenses interfere with this process and therefore are detrimental to the cornea. Examine the eyes of all unconscious persons for the existence of hard lenses and remove them if found. It is probably best to remove soft lenses also as some are not designed for extended use and may also damage the eye.

Leaving most hard contact lenses in the eyes longer than 12 hours can result in corneal ulceration. While not serious, this can be a very painful experience. At times even an iritis may result. This condition almost always resolves on its own within one day. The history is the major clue that the diagnosis is correct. If the condition failed to clear within 24 hours, other problems should be looked into such as corneal laceration, foreign body, or eye infection. After removal of the contact lens, place cool cloths or ice packs on the eyes. This patient should be evaluated by a physician to confirm the diagnosis. Provide protection from sunlight. Patching both eyes while at rest will be of help. Give aspirin or other pain medication if available. The patient may have pain from the migration of the lens into one of the recesses of the conjunctiva, or possibly only have noted a loss of refractive correction. At times the complaint is a sudden "I have lost my contact lens!" Never forget to look in the eye as the possible hiding spot for the lens. Examine the eye as described in the section on foreign bodies in the eye. When dealing with a hard lens, use topical anesthesia as described if necessary and available. If the lens is loose, slide it over the pupil and allow the patient to remove it as she usually does. If the lens is adherent, rinse with eye irrigation solution or clean water and try again. If a corneal abrasion exists, patch as indicated above after the lens is removed.

The soft lens may generally be squeezed between the fingers and literally "popped" off. A special rubber pincer is sold that can aid in this maneuver. Hard lenses may also be removed with a special rubber suction cup device.

If the patient is unconscious, the hard lens will have to be removed. Lacking the suction cup device there are two different maneuvers that

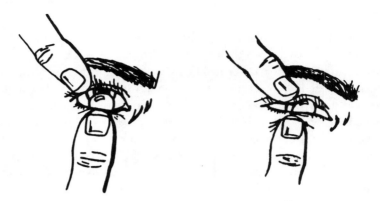

Figure 2-1: Contact lens removal—vertical technique

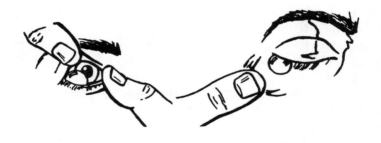

Figure 2-2: Contact lens removal—horizontal technique

may be employed. One is the vertical technique. In this method, move the lens to the center of the eye over the pupil. Then press down on the lower lid, over the lower edge of the contact lens. Next squeeze the eyelids together, thus popping the lens out between them as indicated in figure 2–1. In the horizontal technique, slide the lens to the outside corner of the eye. By tugging on the facial skin near the eye in a downward and outward direction, the lens can pop over the skin edge and be easily removed. See Figure 2–2.

The unconscious patient should have antibiotic salve placed in her eye and the lids taped or patched shut to prevent drying. These patches should be removed when needed for neurological checks, and certainly upon regaining consciousness.

If removal of the lens must be prolonged, safe storage will have to be provided. With regard to hard lenses, the ideal would be marked containers that pad the lenses so that they do not rattle around or otherwise become scratched. Small vials, labeled R and L, filled with a fluff of clean material, taped together and placed in a safe location, would be ideal. Soft contact lenses must be protected from dehydration. It is always proper to store them in normal saline. This solution can be prepared by adding 1½ oz table salt to 1 pint of water. Of course if the patient has a special solution for their lenses in their possession, use it.

Eye Abrasion

Abrasions may be caused by a glancing blow from a wood chip, a swinging branch, even from blowing dirt, embers, ice, or snow. The involved eye should be anesthetized with prescription tetracaine and protected with Tobradex ophthalmic drops. Make sure that a foreign body has not been overlooked.

In cold wind be sure to protect your eyes from the effects of both blowing particles of ice and the wind itself. Grey Owl, in his interesting book, *Tales from an Empty Cabin,* tells how he was walking on one of his long trips through the backwoods along a windswept frozen lake when suddenly he lost sight of the treeline. He felt that he must be in a whiteout, so he turned perpendicular to the wind and hiked toward the shore. Suddenly he bumped into a tree and realized that he was blind! He saved himself only by digging a snow cave and staying put for three days. He wondered how many good woodsmen were lost on their trap lines by such a similar incident, apparently a temporary opacification of the cornea from the cold wind or ice crystal abrasions.

Snow Blindness or Ultraviolet Eye Injury

Snow blindness is a severely painful condition primarily caused by ultraviolet B rays of the sun, which are considerably reflected by snow (85%), water (10-100%), and sand (17%). Thin cloud layers allow the transmission of these rays, while filtering out infra-red (heat) rays of the sun. Thus, it is possible on a rather cool, overcast day with bright snow conditions to become sunburned or snow blind.

Properly approved (ANSI) sunglasses will block 99.8% of the ultraviolet B rays. Suitable glasses should be tagged as meeting these standards.

Non-prescription glasses must be proper fitting and ideally provide side protection. A suitable retention strap must be worn, as I finally learned while rafting on the Green River in Colorado. And for those of us who must learn these things more than once, a second pair of glasses—particularly if prescription lenses are worn—is essential. Lacking sunglasses, any field-expedient method of eliminating glare, such as slit glasses made from wood or any material at hand, including the ubiquitous bandanna, will help. An important aspect of snow blindness is the delayed onset of symptoms. The pain and loss of vision may not be evident until after damaging exposure has been sustained.

Besides snow blindness, either direct or reflected ultraviolet exposure can result in headache or sometimes *Herpes simplex* sores on the lips (see page 57). The headache can be treated with pain medication (see page 30) or look for other underlying causes (see page 34).

Snow blindness is a self limiting affliction. However not only is the loss of vision a problem, but so is the terrible pain, usually described as feeling like red hot pokers were massaging the eye sockets. Lacking any first aid supplies the treatment would be a gentle eye patch and the application of cold packs as needed for pain relief. Generally both eyes are equally affected with a virtual total loss of vision. If there is partial sight and the party is moving, then patching the most affected eye may be practical. Otherwise, rest and patch both eyes.

The prescription tetracaine ophthalmic drops will help ease the pain, but long-term use can delay eye surface healing. Oral pain medication will be of help and should be used. The severe pain can last from hours to several days. In case a drainage of pus or crusting of the eyelids occurs, start antibiotic ophthalmic ointment applications as indicated in the section on conjunctivitis.

Conjunctivitis

Conjunctivitis, an infection or inflammation of the eye surface, will be heralded by a scratchy feeling, almost indistinguishable from a foreign body in the eye. The sclera (white of the eye) will be reddened. Generally the eye will be matted shut in the morning with pus or granular matter.

Infections are generally caused by bacteria, but viral infections also occur. Viral infections tend to have a blotchy red appearance over the white of the eye, while bacterial infections have a generalized red appearance. The drainage in bacterial infections tends to be pus, while virus usually cause a watery discharge.

Allergic conjunctivitis will result in a faint pink coloration and a clear drainage. There are frequently other symptoms of allergy such as runny nose, no fever, and no lymph node enlargement. With either viral or bacterial conjunctivitis, look for fever and possibly lymph node enlargement in the neck. Runny nose and sinus infection are frequently present also. Be sure that a foreign body is not the cause of the reddish eye and infection. If so, it must be removed.

Rinse with clean water frequently during the day. Eye infections such as common bacterial conjunctivitis, the most common infection, are self limiting and will generally clear themselves within two weeks. They can become much worse, however, so medical attention should be sought. Do not patch, but protect the eyes from sunlight. When one eye is infected, treat both eyes as the infection spreads easily to the non-infected eye. There is no suitable non-prescription medication, but note the discussion concerning the use of non-Rx Neosporin or Polysporin in the section on eye foreign body removal. From the Rx supplies one could use the Tobradex ophthalmic drops 3 times a day for 5 to 7 days. If the infection fails to show improvement within 48 hours, probably the antibiotic will not be effective. Reasons for antibiotic failure include: a missed foreign body, allergy to the antibiotic or to something else such as pollen, or resistance of an infectious germ to the antibiotic being used. Switch medications in the case of no improvement after 48 hours. When no other antibiotic ointment is available, use oral antibiotic such as doxycycline 100 mg, 1 capsule twice daily or the alternative antibiotics suggested for the Rx Oral/Topical Module. If the eye is improving, continue use as indicated above, continuing for a full 24 hours after symptoms have ceased.

Iritis

Iritis is an inflammatory disease of the eye having the general appearance of conjunctivitis, but while in the latter the reddish color fades to white near the iris of the eye (the colored part), with iritis the rim of sclera (white of the eye) around the iris is more inflamed or reddened than the white portion further out. The pupil will not constrict when light is shined at it. Provide sun protection. Give aspirin or other pain medication if available. This patient requires urgent evacuation to a specialist. The non-Rx treatment will consist of giving the patient ibuprofen 800 mg every 6 hours. Provide sun protection. Use the Rx

Lorcet 10/650, 1 tablet every 4 hours for pain relief. Instill Tobradex ophthalmic drops four times a day.

As iritis progresses, the red blush near the iris will become more pronounced and a spasm of the muscle used in operation of the iris will cause the pupil to become irregular. With further progression, it is possible for the pupil (anterior chamber) to become cloudy, for cataracts and glaucoma to develop, and serious scarring of eye tissues to develop. Sometimes a profound conjunctivitis or corneal abrasion will cause an iritis that will clear as the problem clears. Some cases of mild iritis can be cleared with agents that dilate the pupil without steroid use. All cases of iritis require treatment by an ophthalmologist.

Allergic Conjunctivitis

The common wilderness causes of *allergic conjunctivitis* are sensitivity to inhaled pollens and irritation from wood smoke. This problem is usually associated with a runny nose (rhinitis) and at times swelling of the eyelids. Rarely there will be a generalized skin itching and the appearance of welts (urticaria). In severe cases there can be considerable swelling of the conjunctival covering of the white of the eye (sclera), forming what appears as fluid-filled sacs over the sclera of the eye (but not covering the cornea). This puffy tissue generally has a light pink tinge to it. While this can look terrible, it is not serious and will resolve on its own within 48 hours, after further exposure to the causative agent ceases.

From the non-Rx supplies give Percogesic 1 tablet 4 times a day and use the tetrahydrozoline eye drops, 2 in each eye every 3 or 4 hours as needed. Percogesic is used for its decongestant actions, and it will also treat the itchy discomfort of this condition. Incidentally, neither of these uses are indicated on the product label.

Sties and Chalazia

The infections of the eyelid called *sties* and *chalazia* can cause scratching of the cornea surface. Often the victim thinks that something is in the eye when, in fact, one of these small pimples is forming. The sty is an infection along a hair follicle on the eyelid margin. The chalazion is an infection of an oil gland on the inner lid margin. The patient will have redness, pain, and swelling along the edge of the upper or lower eyelid. At times the eye will be red with evidence of infection, or conjunctivitis. An eyelid may be swollen, without the pimple formation, when this problem first develops. There should not be extensive swelling around the eye. That could represent a periorbital cellulitis, which is a serious infection requiring treatment with injectable antibiotics. Make sure that a foreign body is not causing the symptoms. Check the eye and eyelids as indicated in that section. While so checking, ascertain if there is a pimple formation that confirms the diagnosis. If it is on the upper lid and it is scratching the eye while blinking, patch the eye and send to a physician for treatment. If no medical care is available, have the patient place warm compresses on the eye for 20 minutes every 2 hours to cause the sty to come to a head. When it does, it may spontaneously break and drain. If it does not drain in two days, open it with a flick of a sharp blade or needle. Continue the warm compresses and provide medication as below. If Rx supplies are available, instill Tobradex ophthalmic drops 3 times a day. (Also note discussion concerning the use of over-the-counter antibiotic ointment in the eye on page 38.) If the lid is quite swollen, give the patient doxycycline 100 mg twice daily or Levaquin 500 mg once daily. Once localized and draining, the oral antibiotic will not be necessary.

Spontaneous Subconjunctival Hemorrhage

This condition, an amazingly common problem, presents as bright bleeding over a portion of the white of the eye. (Actually a hemorrhage has occurred between the white of the eye and the mucus membrane covering it.) It spreads out over a period of 12 to 48 hours, then re-absorbs slowly over the next 7 to 21 days, next turning the conjunctiva yellowish as the blood is reabsorbed. There should not be any pain with this condition, although some people may report a vague "full" feeling in the eye. It normally occurs without cause, but can appear after blunt trauma, or violent coughing, sneezing, or vomiting. No treatment is necessary and evacuation is not required unless associated with trauma.

Blunt Trauma to the Eye

The immediate treatment is to immobilize the injured eye as soon as possible by patching both eyes and moving the patient only by litter. Double vision could mean that there has been a fracture of the skull near the eye or that a problem has developed within the central nervous system. Double vision is sometimes caused by swelling of tissue behind the eyelid. A hyphema may appear, which is a collection of blood in the anterior chamber of the eye. The blood settles in front of the pupil, behind the cornea, and can settle with a distinct blood fluid level becoming easily noticed simply by looking carefully at the pupil and iris.

Patch as indicated in the section on serious injury eye-patch techniques. Patients with hyphema and serious blunt trauma should be evacuated to a physician for care. Have the patient sit with head up, from 45° to 90° to allow blood to pool at the lower edge of the anterior chamber. Check the eye twice daily for drainage, which might indicate infection. If infection develops, treat with oral antibiotic such as the doxycycline 100 mg twice daily. The Tobradex ophthalmic drops may be instilled three times daily. Treat with oral pain medications such as the Lorcet 10/650 1 tablet every 4 hours. Give Atarax 25 mg 4 times daily as needed to potentiate the pain medication and help alleviate nausea or 50 mg 4 times daily if required to calm the patient.

Provide the strongest pain medications required to prevent the injured patient from grimacing and squeezing the injured eye, so as not to compromise the eye contents even more. Small corneal or scleral lacerations may require no treatment at all, but these should be seen and evaluated by a physician if at all possible. Note that severe injury to one eye may even cause blindness to develop in the other eye due to "sympathetic ophthalmia," which is probably an allergic response to eye pigment of the injured eye entering the victim's blood stream.

Glaucoma

Glaucoma is the rise of pressure within the eyeball (intra-ocular pressure increase). The most common form (open angle glaucoma) generally is not encountered before the age of 40. The patient notes halos around lights, mild headaches, loss of vision to the sides (peripheral field cuts), and loss of ability to see well at night. The external eye usually appears normal. This frequently affects both eyes. This condition is generally of gradual onset so that the patient can consult a physician upon returning from the bush.

Initial treatment is with a prescription drug, one drop of 0.5% pilocarpine. It would not be necessary to carry this particular medication, except to treat this condition. This problem should be detected by the pre-trip physical examination. Everyone over the age of 40 should have their intra-ocular pressure tested prior to departure.

Acute glaucoma (narrow angle glaucoma) is much less common than open angle glaucoma, but is much more spectacular in onset. Acute glaucoma is characterized by a rapid rise in pressure of the fluid within the eyeball, causing blurred vision, severe pain in the eye, and even abdominal distress from vagal nerve stimulation. An acute attack can sometimes be broken with pilocarpine, but often needs emergency surgery. A thorough eye examination should be done before the trip to discover those eyes with narrow angles that could result in acute glaucoma. In eyes likely to develop acute glaucoma, a laser iridectomy can be done as an outpatient to prevent an acute narrow angle glaucoma attack.

Events that might precipitate an acute glaucoma attack can include the use of certain medications, such as decongestants. If anyone develops severe eye pain while taking a decongestant or other non-essential medication, have them stop taking it immediately. Severe eye pain from any cause is a reason for urgent evacuation of the patient.

Nose

Nasal Congestion

Nasal congestion is caused by an allergic reaction to pollen, dust, or other allergens, and viral or bacterial upper respiratory infections. Bacterial infections can be cured with antibiotics, but otherwise all are treated similarly for symptomatic relief. Use Percogesic, 1 tablet every 6 hours as needed for nasal congestion or discomfort. Drink lots of liquid to prevent the mucous from becoming too thick. Thick mucous will not drain well and can pack the sinus cavities with increasingly painful pressure.

If the patient has no fever, do not give an antibiotic. A low grade temperature is probably viral and still does not warrant an antibiotic. If a temperature greater than 101° F (38° C) is present, then treat with antibiotic such as the doxycycline 100 mg twice daily or the Zithromax as indicated on page 222.

Foreign Body Nose Injury

Foul drainage from one nostril may well indicate a foreign body. In adults the history of something being placed up the nose would, of course, help in the diagnosis. In a child drainage from one nostril must be considered to be a foreign body until ruled out. Have the patient try to blow his nose to remove the foreign body. With an infant it may be possible for a parent to gently puff into the baby's mouth to force the object out of the nose. While having a nasal speculum would be ideal, any instrument that can be used to spread the nostrils open will work, for example, the pliers on your Swiss Army knife or Leatherman tool. Spread the tips apart after placing them just inside the nostril. One can stretch the nostril quite extensively without causing pain. Shine a light into the nostril passage and attempt to spot the foreign body. Try to grasp the object with another forceps or other instrument. If the foreign material is loose debris—a capsule that broke in the patient's mouth and was sneezed into the nostrils—it is best to irrigate this material out rather than attempting to cleanse with a Q-tip, etc. Place a bulb or irrigation syringe in the clear nostril. With the patient repeating an "eng" sound, flush water, and hopefully the debris, out the opposite nostril.

After removing a foreign body, be sure to check the nostril again for an additional one. Try not to push a foreign body down the back of the patient's throat where he may choke on it. If this is unavoidable, have the patient bend over, with the face down, to decrease the chance of choking. After pushing the object further into the nose and into the upper part of the pharynx, hopefully the victim can cough the object out. If you are using this technique, first read the sections on *nose bleed* and the *Heimlich maneuver.*

Nose Bleed

If nose bleeding (epistaxis) is caused from a contusion to the nose, the bleeding is usually self-limited. Bleeding that starts without trauma is generally more difficult to stop. Most bleeding is from small arteries located near the front of the nose partition, or nasal septum. The best treatment is direct pressure. Have the victim squeeze the nose between her fingers for ten minutes by the clock (a very long time when there is no clock to watch). If this fails, squeeze another ten minutes. Do not blow the nose for this will dislodge clots and start the bleeding all over again. If the bleeding is severe, have the victim sit up to prevent choking on blood and to aid in the reduction of the blood pressure in the nose. Cold compresses do little good.

Continued bleeding can result in shock. This will in turn decrease the bleeding. The sitting position is mandatory to prevent choking on blood from a severe bleed and, as indicated above, will aid in the reduction of blood pressure in the nose. Taken to the extreme degree this position aids in allowing shock to occur.

Another technique that can be tried is to wet a gauze strip thoroughly with the epinephrine from the syringe in the Anakit or Anaguard, a component of the prescription medical kit. The epinephrine can act as a vaso-constrictor to decrease the blood flow and allow clotting. Those having only non-prescription medical supplies will have to use the tetrahyrozoline eye drops, which will not be as powerful in their action. First clear the nose of blood clot so the gauze can be in direct contact with the nasal membranes. Have the victim blow his nose or use the irrigation syringe. Place the epinephrine-soaked gauze in the nose and apply pinching pressure. Pinch for ten minute increments. The gauze may be removed after the bleeding has stopped.

Nose Fracture

A direct blow causing a nasal fracture (broken nose) is associated with pain, swelling, and nasal bleeding. The pain is usually point tender, which means that a very light touch elicits pain, indicating that a fracture has occurred at that location. While the bleeding from trauma to the nose can initially be intense, it seldom lasts more than a few minutes. Apply a cold compress, or a damp cloth that can cool by evaporative cooling. Allow the patient to pinch his nose to aid in reducing bleeding.

If the nose is laterally displaced (shoved to one side), push it back into place. More of these fractures have been treated by coaches on the playing field than have been reduced by doctors. If it is a depressed fracture, a specialist will have to properly elevate the fragments. As soon as the person returns from the bush, have him seen by a physician, but this is not a reason for expensive urgent evacuation. Provide pain medication, but this should only be necessary for a few doses. It is rare to need to pack a bleeding nose due to trauma and this should be avoided, if possible, due to the increased pain it would cause.

Ear

Problems with the ear involve pain, loss of hearing, or drainage. Traumas involving the ear could include lacerations, blunt trauma and hemorrhage (bleeding) in the outer ear tissue, damage from pressure changes of the eardrum (barotrauma) from diving, high altitude, explosions, or direct blows to the ear. See Table 2–5 for signs and symptoms.

Earache

Pain in the ear can be associated with a number of sources, as indicated in Table 2–5. The history of trauma will be an obvious source of pain as mentioned. Most ear pain is due to an *otitis media,* infection behind the eardrum (tympanic membrane), or to *otitis externa,* infection in the outer ear canal (auditory canal). It can also be caused by infection elsewhere (generally a dental infection, infected tonsil, or lymph node in

Table 2-5

Symptoms and Signs of Ear Pathology

	Hearing Loss	Pain	Head Congestion	Ear	Fever
Drainage					
Trauma	■	■		●	
Foreign Body		●		●	
Infection:					
Inner ear	■	■	■	*	■
outer ear	●	●	■		●
Allergy	●	●	■		
Dental source		■			
TMJ source		●			
Lymph node source		●			

Legend:
■	A frequent or intense symptom
●	Common, less intense symptom
Blank	Less likely to produce this symptom

* Only if the eardrum ruptures will drainage occur in an inner ear infection. After the rupture, the pain decreases remarkably.

the neck near the ear). Allergy can result in pressure behind the ear drum and is also a common source of ear pain.

In the bush a simple physical examination and the additional medical history will readily (and generally accurately) distinguish the difference between an otitis media or otitis externa, and sources of pain beyond the ear. Pushing on the nob at the front of the ear (the tragus) or pulling on the ear lobe will elicit pain with an otitis externa. This will not hurt if the patient has otitis media. The history of head congestion favors otitis media. A swollen tender nodule in the neck near the ear would be an infected lymph node. If the skin above the swelling is red, the patient probably has an infected skin abscess. The pain from an abscess is so localized that confusion with an ear infection is seldom a problem. (Refer to *abscess,* page 115). One or more tender lymph nodes can hurt to the extent that confusion of the exact source of the pain may be in doubt. Swollen, tender lymph nodes in the neck are usually associated with pharyngitis (sore throat), with severe otitis externa, or with infections of the skin in the scalp. The latter should be readily noted by examination—palpate the scalp for infected cysts or abscesses. Dental caries, or cavities, can hurt to the extent that the pain seems to come from the ear. They can ordinarily be identified during a careful examination of the mouth. If an obvious cavity is not visualized with a light, try tapping on each tooth to see if pain is suddenly elicited. (See *dental caries*, page 59).

Outer Ear Infection

Outer ear infection of the auditory canal (otitis externa), the part of the ear that opens to the outside, is commonly called "swimmer's ear." The external auditory canal generally becomes inflamed from conditions of high humidity, accumulation of ear wax, or contact with contaminated water. Scratching the ear after picking the nose or scratching elsewhere may also be a source of this common infection.

Prevent cold air from blowing against the ear. Warm packs against the ear or instilling comfortably warm sweet oil or even cooking oil can help. Provide pain medication. Obtain professional help if the patient develops a fever, the pain becomes severe, or lymph nodes, or adjacent neck tissues start swelling. Significant tissue swelling will require antibiotic treatment. At times a topical ointment will suffice, but with fever, swollen lymph or skin structures an oral antibiotic will be required.

Triple antibiotic ointment with pramoxine from the Topical Bandaging Module will work fine for outer ear infections. This is not approved by the FDA for this use, as ear infections are serious and it is not intended that non-physicians treat this condition without medical help. From the Rx kit, one could use the Tobradex ophthalmic drops. These medications should be applied with the ear facing up and, in the case of the ointment, allowed to melt by body temperature. This may take 5 minutes per ear. Place cotton in the ear to hold the medication in place. Instill medication 4 times daily and treat for 14 days. If the canal is swollen shut, a steroid ointment may also be used in between applications of the other ointments just described. From the Topical Bandaging Module use the hydrocortisone 1% cream in addition to the triple antibiotic ointment. Tobradex contains enough steroid to be adequate for these purposes. Swollen tissue and/or fever also require an oral antibiotic. From the Rx Oral/Topical Medication Module use the doxycycline 100 mg twice daily or the Levaquin 500 mg daily. Provide the best pain medication that you can. From your non-Rx Oral Medication Module use 1 or 2 Percogesic every four hours. From the Rx

Oral/Topical Medication Module give Lorcet 10/650, 1 tablet every 4 hours as needed.

Middle Ear Infection

Middle ear infection (otitis media) presents in a person who has sinus congestion and possibly drainage from allergy or infection. The ear pain can be excruciating. Fever will frequently be intermittent, normal at one moment and over 103° F (39° C) at other times. Fever indicates bacterial infection of the fluid trapped behind the eardrum. If the eardrum ruptures, the pain will cease immediately and the fever will drop. This drainage allows the body to cure the infection, but will result in at least temporary damage to the ear drum and decreased hearing until it heals.

There is no increased pain when pulling on the ear lobe or pushing on the tragus (the nob in front of the ear) in this condition, unless an outer ear infection is also present. If you were to look at the eardrum with an otoscope, it would be red and bulging out from pressure or sucked back by a vacuum in the middle ear.

You do not need an otoscope to diagnose this condition. Many people will complain of hearing loss and think they have wax or a foreign body in the ear canal, when they actually have fluid accumulation behind the eardrum. Consequently, ear drops and washing the ear will not help improve this condition. Beside pain, the key to the diagnosis is head congestion and fever.

There is little that can be accomplished without medication. Protect the ear from cold, position the head so that the ear is directed upwards, and provide warm packs to the ear. While drops do not help cure this problem, some pain relief may be obtained with warmed sweet oil (or even cooking oil) drops in the ear.

Treatment will consist of providing decongestant, pain medication, and oral antibiotic. A good decongestant and pain reliever from the non-Rx Oral Medication kit is Percogesic, 2 tablets 4 times daily. Rx pain medication is given as needed, as indicated in the previous section. Only the Rx Oral/Topical Module has the proper antibiotics to treat this condition. Use doxycycline 1 tablet twice daily or Levaquin 500 mg daily, generally for 5 to 7 days.

If the pressure causes the ear drum to rupture, the pain and fever will cease, but there will be a bloody drainage from the ear. Hearing is always decreased with the infection and will remain decreased due to the ruptured eardrum for some time. This generally heals itself quite well, but treat with decongestant to decrease the drainage and allow the eardrum to heal. Avoid placing drops or ointments in the ear canal if there is a chance that the eardrum has ruptured, as many medications are damaging to the inner ear mechanisms.

Foreign Body Ear Injury

These are generally of three types: accumulation of wax plugs (cerumen), foreign objects, and living insects. Wax plugs can usually be softened with a warmed oil. This may have to be placed in the ear canal repeatedly over many days. Irrigating with room temperature water may be attempted with a bulb syringe, such as the one recommended for wound irrigation in the Topical Bandaging Module. If a wax-plugged ear becomes painful, treat as indicated in the section on otitis externa.

The danger in trying to remove inanimate objects is the tendency to shove them further into the ear canal or to damage the delicate ear canal lining, thus adding bleeding to your troubles. Of course, rupturing the eardrum by shoving against it would be a real unnecessary disaster. Attempt to grasp a foreign body with a pair of tweezers if you can see it. Do not poke blindly with anything. Irrigation may be attempted as indicated above. A popular method of aiding in the management of insects in the ear canal is the instillation of lidocaine to kill the bug instantly, prior to attempting removal. There are reports of lidocaine making a person very dizzy, especially if it leaks through a hole in the eardrum into the inner ear. This dizziness is very distressing and may result in profound vomiting and discomfort. It is self-limiting, however, and should not last more than a day if it does transpire. An alternate method is to drown the bug with cooking or other oil, then attempt removal. Oil seems to kill bugs quicker than water. The less struggle, the less chance for stinging, biting, or other trauma to the delicate ear canal and eardrum. Tilt the ear downward, thus hoping to slide the dead bug towards the entrance where it can be grappled. Shining a light at the ear to coax a bug out is probably futile.

Ruptured Eardrum

Rupture of the eardrum (tympanic membrane perforation) can result from direct puncture, from explosions, and from the barotrauma of diving deep or rapid ascent to high altitude. Being smacked on the ear can also rupture the eardrum.

Avoid diving or rapid ascents of altitude in vehicles or airplanes if suffering from sinus congestion. Congestion can lead to blockage of the eustachian tube. Failure to equilibrate pressure through this tube be-tween the middle ear and the throat, and thus the outside world, can re-sult in damage to the eardrum. In case of congestion, take a decongestant and pain medication combination such as Percogesic 2 tablets every 4 hours until clear. Cancel any plans of diving if congested. Also, if a gradual pressure squeeze is causing pain while diving, the dive should be terminated.

When flying, it will be noted that blocked eustachian tubes will cause more pain upon descent than ascent. When going up the pressure in the inner ear will increase and blow out through the eustachian tube. When coming down increased outer atmospheric pressure is much less apt to clear the plugged tube and a squeeze of air against the eardrum will re-sult. Try to equalize this pressure by pinching the nose shut and gently increasing the pressure in your mouth and throat against closed lips. This will generally clear the eustachian tube and relieve the air squeeze on the eardrum. Do not overdo this; that can also be painful. If barotrauma results in eardrum rupture, the pain should instantly cease. There may be bloody drainage from the ear canal. Do not place drops in the ear canal, but drainage can be gently wiped away or frequently changed cotton plugs used to catch the bloody fluid.

Temporal–Mandibular–Joint Syndrome

TMJ syndrome is actually a problem of the jaw, but the pain radiates into the ear so often, that we will consider it primarily as a source of ear pain. The temporal-mandibular joint is the hinge joint of the jaw, lo-cated just forward of the ear. You can easily feel it move if you place a finger tip into your ear canal. When this joint becomes inflamed, it will frequently cause ear pain. It will then be painful to fingertip pressure di-rectly on the joint. No swelling should be noted. Tenderness is increased with chewing, and pain and popping or locking may be noted when opening the jaw widely. The pain radiates into the temple area and when severe, the entire head hurts.

Treatment is with local heat. The use of ibuprofen or Percogesic can be very helpful. At times Lorcet 10/650, 1 tablet every 4 hours, may be required. Do not eat foods that are hard to chew or that require opening the mouth widely.

Mouth and Throat

Sore Throat

The most common cause of a sore throat, or pharyngitis, is a viral infection. While uncomfortable, this malady requires no antibiotic treatment—in fact, antibiotics will do no good whatsoever. Strictly speaking, the only sore throat that needs to be treated is the one caused by a specific bacteria (beta hemolytic streptococcus, Lancefield group A) as it has been found that antibiotic treatment for 10 days will avoid the dreaded complication of rheumatic fever, which may occur in 1 to 3% of the people who contract this particular infection. Many purists in the medical profession feel that no antibiotics should be used until the results of a throat culture or antibody screen proving this particular infection have been returned from the lab. On a short trip the victim can be taken to a doctor for a strep culture to determine if the sore throat was indeed strep. On a wilderness trip longer than 2 weeks, it would be best to commit the patient to a 10-day therapy of antibiotics, realizing that the symptoms will soon pass and the patient seem well, but that it is essential to continue the medication for the full 10 days.

There are textbook differences in the general appearance of a viral and strep sore throat. The lymph nodes in the neck are swollen in both cases; they are more tender with bacterial infections, but people with a low pain threshold will complain bitterly about soreness regardless of the source of infection. The throat will be quite red in bacterial infection and a white splotchy coating over the red tonsils or back portion of the throat generally means a strep infection—at least these classic indications are present 20% of the time. Sore throats caused by some viral infections (namely infectious mononucleosis and adenovirus) may mimic all of the above. From the Rx Oral/Topical Medication Module use Zithromax 500 mg as described. The 6 tablet dose provides a therapeutic blood level for 10 days.

Infectious Mononucleosis

Infectious mononucleosis, a disease of young adults (teens through 30 years of age) generally presents as a terrible sore throat, swollen lymph nodes (normally at the back of the neck and not as tender as with strep infection), and a profound feeling of fatigue. It is self-limited with total recovery to be expected after 2 weeks for most victims—some, unfortunately are bedridden for weeks and lethargic for 6 months. Spleen enlargement is common. The most serious aspect of this disease is the possibility of splenic rupture, but this is rare. Avoid palpating the spleen (shoving on the left upper quadrant of the abdomen), let the victim rest, no hiking, etc., until the illness and feeling of lethargy has passed. The first 5 days are the worst, with fever and excruciating sore throat being the major complaint.

Treatment is symptomatic with medication for fever and pain such as the non-Rx Percogesic or ibuprofen each given 1 or 2 tablets every 4 to 6 hours, or the Rx Lorcet 10/650 1 tablet every 4 to 6 hours. A mild form of hepatitis frequently occurs with mononucleosis that causes nausea and loss of appetite. This requires no specific treatment other than rest. If severe ear pain begins, add a decongestant (or just use the Percogesic) 1 tablet every 6 hours to promote relief of eustachian tube pressure. Due to the uncertainty of diagnosis, treat the severe sore throat as if it were a strep infection with antibiotic for 10 days or the Zithromax as indicated above.

Mouth Sores

When mouth sores develop patients frequently believe they either have cancer or infection, especially herpes. A common reason for a lesion is the sore called a papilloma, caused from rubbing against a sharp tooth or dental work. They may look serious but are not. They are raised, normally orange in color. One can usually find an obvious rough area causing the irritation. Treatment is to avoid chewing at the lesion and to apply 1% hydrocortisone cream from the Topical Bandaging Module every 3 hours. If the Rx Oral/Topical Module is available, use the Topicort .25% ointment every 4 hours. An alternative therapy, which can be used simultaneously, is to apply oil of cloves (eugenol).

A *canker sore,* also called an aphthous ulcer, can appear anywhere in the mouth and be any size. It has a distinctive appearance of a white crater with a red, swollen border. Treatment is as above.

If there is generalized tissue swelling, possibly drainage or whitish cover on the gums, foul-smelling breath, and gums and mouth tissue that bleeds easily when scraped, it is possible that the victim has trench mouth or Vincent's infection. This is caused by poor hygiene, which is unfortunately common on long expeditions under adverse circumstances. If the white exudate is located over the tonsils, one has to be concerned about strep throat (see page 55), mononucleosis (see page 55), and diphtheria (see page 236). Treat trench mouth with warm water rinses, swishing the crud off as well as possible. If the Rx Oral/Topical

Medication Module is available, give the full dose regimen of Zithromax or treat with Levaquin 500 mg once daily for 4 to 5 days.

The mouth lesions of herpes simplex begin as small blisters and leave a raw area once they have broken open. The ulceration from a herpes is red rather than the white of the canker sore. They are very painful. From the Rx Oral/Topical Module apply the Denavir cream every two hours. This is not approved for use inside of the mouth, but it is perfectly safe and it works.

Fever blisters are sores that break out on the vermillion border of the lips, generally as a result of herpes simplex virus eruptions. These lesions can be activated by fevers (hence their name "fever blister"), or other trauma, even mental stress. Ultraviolet light will frequently cause flares of fever blisters. This can be a common problem of mountain travel due to the more intense UV radiation encountered at higher altitudes. Treat as above for the herpes simplex inner mouth lesions. These lesions can be prevented with adequate sunscreen and/or by taking an anti-viral such as Zovirax capsules, 400 mg twice daily.

Gum Pain or Swelling

Pain attended by swelling high on the gum at the base of the tooth usually indicates an infection and a tooth that may require extraction, or root canal therapy, if a dentist can be consulted who has brought more than just his fly rod with him on the trip. Attempting to treat without either option, have the patient use warm water mouth rinses. Start the victim on antibiotics as indicated in the previous section. If a bulging area can be identified in the mouth, an incision into the swollen gum with a sharp blade may promote drainage. If the pain is severe and not relieved with the Rx Lorcet 10/650, or any other pain medication that you have, the tooth may have to be pulled.

Swelling at the gumline, rather than at the base of the tooth, may indicate a periodontal abscess. The gingiva (or gums) are red, swollen, foul smelling and oozing. Frequently this represents food particle entrapment and abscess formation along the surface of the tooth with the gums, the so-called gingival cuff. Considerable relief can often be obtained by probing directly into the abscess area through the gingival cuff, using any thin, blunt instrument. Probe along the length of the tooth to break up and drain the abscess. Have the patient use frequent hot mouth rinses to continue the drainage process. If a foreign object, such as a piece of food, is causing the swelling, irrigate with warm salt solution or warm water, with sufficient force to dislodge the particle. Probe it loose if necessary. Dental floss may be very helpful.

Acute pain and swelling of the tissue behind the third molar usually represents an erupting wisdom tooth. Technically this is called "pericoronitis." There is a little flap of tissue that lies over the erupting wisdom tooth called the *operculum*. Biting on this causes it to swell, and then it becomes much easier to bite on it again, and so on. The end result is considerable pain. This can be relieved by surgically removing the operculum. If local anesthetic is available, such as lidocaine, inject it directly into the operculum and then cut it out with a sharp blade using the outline of the erupting tooth as a guideline. The bleeding can soon be stopped by biting down on a gauze or other cloth after the procedure is over. Stitching this wound is not required. If no lidocaine is available, swab the area with alcohol as this helps provide some slight anesthesia. Application of powder from an opened diphenhydramine capsule from the Non-Rx Oral Medication Module might provide some anesthesia.

Swelling of the entire side of the face will occur with dental infections that spread. This condition should ideally be treated in a hospital with intravenous antibiotics. In the bush apply warm compresses to the face. Do not lance the infection from the skin side, but a peaked, bulging area on the inside of the mouth may be lanced to promote drainage. Abscess extension into surrounding facial tissues generally means that lancing will do little good. This patient is very ill and rest is mandatory. Provide antibiotic coverage from the Rx Oral/Topical Medication Module with Levaquin 500 mg once daily, the Zithromax as indicated on page 57, or from the Rx Injectable Medication Module the Rocephin giving 500 mg by intramuscular injection every 12 hours.

Mouth Lacerations

Any significant trauma to the mouth causes considerable bleeding and concern. The bleeding initially always seems worse than it is. Rinse the mouth with warm water to clear away the clots so that you can identify the source of the bleeding.

Laceration of the piece of tissue that seems to join the bottom lip or upper lip to the gum line is a common result of trauma to the mouth and need not be repaired, even though it initially looks horrible and may bleed considerably. This is called the labial frenum. Simply stuff some gauze into the area until the bleeding stops.

A laceration of the tongue will not require stitching (suturing) unless an edge is deeply involved. Fairly deep cuts along the top surface and bottom can be ignored in the wilderness setting. If suturing is to be accomplished and you have injectable lidocaine from the Rx Injectable Module, inject into the lower gum behind the teeth on the side of the gum facing the tongue. Technically this area is called the median raphe distal to the posterior teeth. This will block the side of the tongue and be much less painful than directly injecting into the tongue. Use the 3-0 gut sutures. These sutures will dissolve within a few days. Sutures in the tongue frequently come out within a few hours, even when they are well tied, much to the victim and surgeon's annoyance. If this happens and the tongue is not bleeding badly, just leave it alone. Minor cuts along the edge of the tongue can also be ignored.

Make sure that cuts on the inside of the mouth do not have foreign bodies, such as pieces of tooth inside of them. These must be removed. Inject the lidocaine into the wound before probing if you have the Rx Injectable Medication Module. Irrigate thoroughly with water. Even without the lidocaine, the inside of the mouth can be stitched with minimal pain. Use the 3-0 gut suture, removing them in 4 days if they have not fallen out already. Refer to page 100 for discussion of suturing the face and the outside portion of the lips.

Dental Pain

Cavities may be identified by visual examination of the mouth in most cases. At times the pain is so severe that the patient cannot tell exactly which tooth is the offender. It helps to know that: a painful tooth will not refer pain to the opposite side of the mouth and painful back teeth normally do not refer pain to front teeth and vice-versa. With the painful area narrowed down, look for an obvious cavity. If none is found, tap each tooth in turn until the offending one is reached—a tap on it will elicit strong pain.

Dry the tooth and try to clean out any cavity found. For years oil of cloves, or eugenol, has been used to deaden dental pain. Avoid trying to apply an aspirin directly to a painful tooth; it will only make a worse mess of things. Many excellent dental kits are now available without prescription that contain topical anesthetic agents and temporary fillings. A daub of topical anesthetic will work. In your Topical Bandaging Module you have triple antibiotic with pramoxine that you can use. It's the pramaxine component that provides the pain relief. Before applying the anesthetic, dry the tooth and try to clean out any cavity found. From the Rx Oral/Topical Medication Module, Lorcet 10/650 1 tablet every 4 hours will generally eliminate the most severe dental pain. Or from the Non-Rx Oral Medication Module, give Percogesic 2 tablets every 4 hours for pain. When in the bush and a toothache begins, I would also start treating with an antibiotic if the Rx kit is available. Give Levaquin 500 mg once daily until swelling or pain resolves, which indicates the infection is under control.

Lost Filling

This could turn into a real disaster. An old-fashioned remedy uses powdered zinc oxide (not the ointment) and eugenol. Starting with the two in equal parts, mix until a putty is formed by adding more zinc oxide powder as necessary. This always takes considerably more of the zinc oxide than at first would seem necessary. Pack this putty into the cavity and allow to set over the next 24 hours.

The Cavit dental filling paste in the Rx Oral/Topical Module provides a strong temporary filling. Dry the cavity bed thoroughly with a gauze square. Place several drops of anesthetic, such as oil of cloves (eugenol), to deaden the nerve endings and kill bacteria. The triple antibiotic with pramoxine ointment from the Non-Rx Oral Module can also be used for this purpose. Plain triple antibiotic ointment will not work. You will have to pack the ointment into the cavity area and allow it to melt. Dry the cavity carefully once again. The Cavit paste should be applied to the dry cavity and packed firmly into place. Obviously avoid biting on the side of the filling, regardless of the materials used to make your temporary filling. See a dentist as soon as possible as the loss of a filling may indicate extension of decay in the underlying tooth.

Loose or Dislodged Tooth

When you examine a traumatized mouth and find a tooth that is rotated, or dislocated in any direction, do not push the tooth back into place. Further movement may disrupt the tooth's blood and nerve supply. If the tooth is at all secure leave it alone. The musculature of the lips and tongue will generally gently push the tooth back into place and keep it there.

A fractured tooth with exposed pink substance that is bleeding is showing exposed nerve. This tooth will need protection with eugenol and temporary filling as indicated above. This is actually a dental emergency that should be treated by a dentist immediately.

If a tooth is knocked out, replace it into the socket immediately. If this cannot be done, have the victim hold the tooth under their tongue or in their lower lip until it can be implanted. In any case speed is a matter of great importance. A tooth left out too long will be rejected by the body as a foreign substance.

All of the above problems will mean that a soft diet and avoidance of chewing with the affected tooth for many days will be necessary. In the wilderness setting, start the patient on antibiotic such as the doxycycline 100 mg, 1 daily for any of the above problems.

Trauma that can cause any of the above may also result in fractures of the tooth below the gum line and of the alveolar ridge affecting several teeth. If this is suspected, start the patient on antibiotic as mentioned in the paragraph above. Oral surgical help must be obtained as soon as possible. A soft diet is essential until healing takes place, possibly a matter of 6 to 8 weeks.

Pulling a Tooth

It is best not to pull a tooth from an infected gum, as this might spread the infection. If an abscess is forming, place the patient on antibiotic, such as Levaquin 500 mg daily or doxycycline 100 mg twice daily, and use warm mouth rinses to promote drainage. After the infection has subsided, it is safer to pull the tooth. Opening the abscess as described in *dental abscess* on page 57 will be helpful at times. If it appears necessary to pull an infected tooth, give the patient an antibiotic pill about 2 hours before pulling the tooth to provide some protection against spreading the infection. Pull the tooth by obtaining a secure hold with the universal side-cutting rongeur. (Figure 58) Slowly apply pressure in a back-and-forth, side-to-side motion to rock the tooth free. This loosens the tooth in its socket and will permit its removal. Avoid jerking or pulling the tooth with a straight outward force; it can resist all of the strength that you have in this direction. Jerking may break off the root. The rongeur will grip the tooth surface by cutting into the enamel, holding better than even dental extraction forceps.

If the root breaks off, you may leave it alone rather than trying to dig it out. If the root section is obviously loose, then you can pick it out with some suitable instrument. Thin fragments of bone may fracture off during the extraction. These will work their way to the surface during healing. Do not attempt to replace them, but pick them free as they surface.

If you do not have the side-cutting dental rongeurs or dental forceps, it is best not to attempt to pull the tooth with another instrument. Pliers may crush the tooth and the tooth can slip in your grasp. However, even a large, solid tooth can be removed by using your finger to rock it back and forth. This may take days to accomplish, but it will eventually loosen sufficiently to remove.

Chest

One of the most common reasons for a visit to a physician's office or emergency department is a problem with the chest. Chest pain and shortness of breath can be symptoms of serious disorders and cannot be taken lightly. Fortunately most times the chest pain is benign, generally due to muscle spasm. It can be very difficult to evaluate, even at the emergency department. Chest problems are best evaluated by a physician, but in a remote area, try to sort out your options with the table on page 17. In case of trauma, the patient may have suffered torn muscles between the ribs or broken ribs (see page 151).

Bronchitis/Pneumonia

Infection of the airways in the lung (bronchitis) or infection in the air sacks of the lung (pneumonia) will cause very high fever, persistent cough frequently producing phlegm stained with blood, and cause prostration of the victim. From the Non-Rx Oral Medication Module treat the fever with Percogesic 2 tablets every 4 hours or ibuprofen 200 mg 2 tablets every 4 hours and the cough with diphenhydramine 25 mg every 4 hours (see page 221). If you have the Rx Oral/Topical Medication Module you may treat sharp pleuritic chest pain with Lorcet 10/650, 1 tablet every 4 to 6 hours. It is also a strong cough suppressant as mentioned on page 223. Cool with a wet cloth over the forehead as needed. Do not bundle the patient with a very high fever as this will drive the temperature only higher. The shivering cold feeling that the patient has is only proof that his thermal control mechanism is out of adjustment; trust the thermometer or the back of your hand to follow the patient's temperature. Encourage the patient to drink fluids, as fever and coughing lead to dehydration. This causes the mucous in the bronchioles to become thick and tenacious. Force fluid to prevent this sputum from plugging up sections of the lung.

Provide antibiotic: from the Rx Oral/Topical Medication Module give the Levaquin 500 mg daily until the fever is broken and for an additional 4 days. Alternately give the Zithromax as directed on page 222. Or from the Rx Injectable Medication Module, you may give Rocephin 500 mg twice daily. Prepare a sheltered camp for the victim as best as circumstances permit. Rest until the fever is broken is essential with or without the availability of antibiotic. Encourage the patient to eat even though very ill people lose their appetites.

Pneumothorax

Even in very healthy young adults and teenagers, it is possible for an air cell of the lung to break for no apparent reason and fill a portion of the chest cavity with air, thus collapsing part of one lung. A minor pneumothorax will also spontaneously take care of itself, with the air being reabsorbed and the lung reexpanding over 3 to 5 days. The classic sign of decreased breath sounds over the area of the collapse with be very difficult for the untrained observer, even with a stethoscope. But listen first to one side of the chest and then the other to see if there is a difference. Part of the difficulty lies in the fact that patients with chest pain do not breathe deeply and all breath sounds are decreased. Other parts of the physical exam are even more subtle. In unexplained severe chest pain in an otherwise healthy individual pneumothorax might be the cause.

Severe pneumothorax will have to be treated by a physician with removal of the trapped air with a large syringe, flutter valve, or by other methods currently employed in a hospital setting. If pain is severe and breathing difficult, the only choice is evacuation of the victim.

From the Non-Rx Oral Medication Module you may give 2 Percogesic for pain every 4 hours or 2 to 4 ibuprofen 200 mg tablets every 6 hours. If you have the Rx Oral/Topical Medication Module, give 1 Lorcet 10/650 every 4 hours. This can be augmented with Atarax 25 mg every 6 hours. It is possible for the pain to be so severe that the use of injectable Nubain or inhaled Stadol will be necessary (see page 31).

Pulmonary Embolus

A pulmonary embolus is a blood clot breaking loose from its point of origin, normally from a leg or pelvic vein, which then lodges in the lung after passing through the heart. When serious this condition appears as shortness of breath, rapid breathing, with a dull substernal chest pain. There may be cough, bloody sputum, fever, and sharp chest pain. A pulmonary embolus can mimic *pneumonia* (page 62) and *high altitude pulmonary edema* (page 208). It can be fatal if an embolus large enough to block off more than 50% of the lung circulation occurs at once. This condition generally resolves within a matter of days. Increased risk is found in older people who have been sitting a long time (such as on plane flights) or anyone immobilized after injury. The only medication in the suggested wilderness medical kit that would be of any help would be the ibuprofen 200 mg given 4 times daily. Stronger doses of this product (up to 800 mg given 4 times daily) or additional pain medication can be given to help with the discomfort. Due to the uncertainty of the diagnosis, treat with antibiotic, such as the Zithromax as described on page 222 or the Levaquin 500 mg once daily until the pain and/or fever resolves and then for an additional 4 days. This would not help a pulmonary embolus, but it would properly treat a pneumonia.

Abdomen

Even with years of clinical experience and unlimited laboratory and x-ray facilities, abdominal pain can be a diagnostic dilemma. How serious is it? Should the trip be terminated and evacuation started or can it be waited out or safely treated in the bush? Or what treatment protocol can be followed by those travelers in isolated areas where there is no chance of rescue?

Abdominal Pain

Any abdominal pain that lasts longer than 24 hours is a cause for concern and professional help should be sought if possible. Diagnosis will be determined from the history (type and severity of pain, location, radiation, when it started), as well as certain aspects of the physical examination and the clinical course that develops. Some of these aspects are summarized in Table 2–6 and in the discussion that follows.

A burning sensation in the middle of the upper part of the abdomen (mid-epigastrium) is probably *gastritis* or stomach irritation. If allowed to persist this can develop into an *ulcer*, a crater eaten into the stomach or duodenal wall. In the latter case the pain may be most notable in the right upper quadrant. For some reason ulcers will sometimes feel better if you press against them with your hand. This supposedly was why Napoleon is seen with his hand inside his jacket in his favorite pose—he was pressing against his abdomen to relieve the pain of an ulcer. Severe, persistent mid-epigastric pain, that is also frequently burning in nature, can be *pancreatitis,* an inflammation of the pancreas. This is a serious problem, but rare. Alcohol consumption can cause pancreatitis, as well as gastritis and ulcer formation. It must be avoided if pain in this area de-

Symptoms and Signs of Abdominal Pathology

Table 2-6

	Burning	Nausea*	Food Related	Diarrhea	Fever
Gastritis/ulcer (page 65)	■	●	■		
Pancreatitis (page 65)	■	●	●		●
Hiatal Hernia (page 65)	■	●			
Gall Bladder (page 66)		■	■		●
Appendicitis (page 66)		●			●
Gastroenteritis (page 68)		■	●	■	●
Diverticulitis (page 70)			●	●	●
Colitis (page 70)				■	
Hepatitis (page 178)		■	●		●
Food Poisoning (page 79)		■		■	■ ●

■   Frequent or intense
●   Usual or less intense
Blank   Less likely to be associated
* See also nausea and vomiting, page 68
Note: Page references are in brackets.

velops. In fact, any food that seems to increase the symptoms should be avoided. Reflux of stomach acid up the esophagus, caused by a *hiatal hernia*—protrusion of a part of the stomach through a hole in the diaphragm through which the esophagus passes—will cause the same symptoms. The reflux also causes the burning pain to radiate up the center of the chest.

Treatment for all of the above is aggressive antacid therapy. These conditions can be made worse by eating spicy food, tomato products, and other foods high in acid content. Milk may temporarily help the burning of an ulcer or gastritis, but may increase the burning sensation later. Avoid any medications containing aspirin and ibuprofen. Acid suppression medication such as Tagamet, Zantac, Pepcid, Axid, Prevacid, and Prilosec help greatly and anyone with a history of these disorders should consider adding such items to the medical kit. There is a concern that these medications can make the user more vulnerable to traveler's diarrhea, cholera, and other infectious disease from which a normal or high stomach acid level might otherwise provide some protection. A safer medication for persons afflicted with heartburn not responsive to antacids, who must travel in a third world situation, would be Carafate taken 1 gram 4 times daily. This is a prescription medication.

Mild nausea may be associated with the above problems, but intense nausea could indicate gastroenteritis and food poisoning (generally these cause significant diarrhea also), hepatitis, and gall bladder disorder.

Gastroenteritis, see page 68

Hepatitis, see page 178

Gall Bladder

Nausea associated with pain in the right upper quadrant of the abdomen may be from a *gall bladder* problem. No burning is associated with gall bladder pain, and this discomfort is typically made worse by eating, sometimes even smelling, greasy foods. While drinking cream or milk would initially help the pain of gastritis or an ulcer, it causes an immediate increase in symptoms if the gall bladder is involved. Treatment is avoidance of fatty foods. Nausea and vomiting can be treated as indicated on page 68. Treat for pain as described on page 30. The onset of fever is an important indication of infection of the blocked gall bladder. *This is a surgical emergency.* Treat with the strongest antibiotic available. If the Rx Injectable Medication Module is available, give Rocephin 500 mg, 2 doses IM immediately, repeated with 2 doses every 12 hours. Lacking that medication, give the Levaquin 500 mg daily. Continue to treat the pain and nausea as required for relief. Offer as much fluid as they can tolerate. Gall bladder disease is more common in overweight people over the age of thirty. It is more common in women.

The possibility of *appendicitis* is a major concern as it can occur in any age group, and that includes healthy wilderness travelers. It is fortunately rare. While surgery is the treatment of choice, probably as many as 70% of people not treated with surgery or antibiotics can survive this problem. The survival rate would be much higher with appropriate IV therapy. Of course, timely surgery provides 100% survival.

The classic presentation of this illness is a vague feeling of discomfort around the umbilicus (navel). Temperature may be low grade, 99.6 to 100° F (37° C) at first. Within a matter of 12 hours the discomfort turns to pain and localizes in the right lower quadrant, most frequently at a point two-thirds of the way between the navel and the very top of the right pelvic bone (anterior-superior iliac crest). Ask the patient two questions: Where did you first start hurting? (belly button); now where do you hurt? (right lower quadrant as described). Those answers mean appendicitis until it is ruled out. It is possible but unusual to have diarrhea with appendicitis. Diarrhea usually means that the patient does not have appendicitis. I find it helpful to ask the patient to walk and to watch how they do it. A person with appendicitis will walk with rather careful, short steps, bent slightly forward in pain. They certainly do not bounce off the examining table and walk down the hall to the bathroom. Anyone with springy steps most likely does not have appendicitis.

Sometimes full laboratory and x-ray facilities can do no better in making this diagnosis. The ultimate answer will come from surgical exploration. If a surgeon has doubts, he might wait, with the patient safely in a hospital or at home under close supervision. But the patient with those symptoms should certainly be taken to a surgeon as soon as possible.

In the examination of the painful abdomen, several maneuvers can indicate the seriousness of the situation. The first is to determine how guarded the area is to palpation. If the patient's stomach is rigid to gentle pushing, this can mean that extreme tenderness and irritation of the peritoneum, or abdominal wall lining, exists. Use only gentle pushing. If there is an area of the abdomen where it does not hurt to push, apply pressure rather deeply. Now, suddenly take your hand away! If pain flares over the area of suspect tenderness, this is called *referred rebound tenderness* and means that the irritation has reached an advanced stage. This person should be evacuated to surgical help at once.

What can you do if you are in the deep bush, say the Back River of Canada, without the faintest hope of evacuating the patient? Move the patient as little as possible. No further prodding of the abdomen should be done, as her only hope is that the appendix will form an abscess that will be walled-off by the bodily defense mechanisms. Give no food. Provide small amounts of water, Gatorade, and fruit drinks as tolerated. With advanced disease the intestines will stop working and the patient will vomit any excess. This will obviously cause a disturbance to the gut and possibly rupture the appendix or the abscess.

Treat for pain, nausea, and with antibiotics as indicated in the paragraph above on gall bladder infection.

The abscess should form 24 to 72 hours following onset of the illness. Many surgeons would elect to open and drain this abscess as soon as the patient is brought to them. Other surgeons feel it is best to leave the patient alone at this time and allow the abscess to continue the walling-off process. They feel there is so much inflammation present, surgery only complicates the situation further. Even without surgery, within 2 to 3 weeks the patient may be able to move with minimal discomfort.

One form of therapy never to be employed when there is a suspicion of appendicitis is a laxative. The action of the laxative may cause disruption of the appendix abscess with resultant generalized peritonitis (massive abdominal infection).

It is currently thought that there is no justification for the prophylactic removal of an appendix in an individual, unless he is planning to move to a very remote area without medical help for an extended period of time and it is known from x-ray that he has a fecolith (or stone) in the colon at the mouth of the appendix. Otherwise, the possible later complications of surgical adhesions may well outweigh the "benefit" of such a procedure.

Vomiting

Nausea and vomiting are frequently caused by infections known as gastroenteritis. Many times these are viral so that antibiotics are of no value. These infections will usually resolve without treatment in 24 to 48 hours. Fever is seldom high, but may briefly be high in some cases. Fever should not persist above 100° F (38° C) longer than 12 hours. Nausea may be treated with diphenhydramine 25 mg every 8 hours from the Non-Rx Oral Medication Module or Atarax 25 mg every 6 hours from the Rx Oral/Topical Medication Module. If the Rx Injectable Medication Module is available, severe nausea and vomiting may be treated with Vistaril 25 to 50 mg every 6 hours given intramuscularly. Vomiting without diarrhea will not require the use of an antibiotic. If the vomiting is caused from severe illness, such as an ear infection, then use of antibiotic to treat the underlying cause is justified.

Nausea induced by high altitude, see page 207.

Nausea associated with jaundice, see *hepatitis*, pages 178 to 180.

Nausea from ingestion of seafood, see *paralytic shellfish poisoning*, page 81; *scromboid poisoning*, page 80; and *ciguatera poisoning*, page 80.

See also *poisoning from plant or food ingestion*, page 79; and *poisoning from ingestion of petroleum products*, page 79.

Motion Sickness

Motion in any vehicle can induce nausea, hence the many etiologies of this disorder, such as sea sickness, air sickness, and the dreaded "tilt-awhirl"-induced vomiting at the amusement park. After being exposed to motion for many days—a long nautical trip or train ride—some people become nauseated when the motion suddenly stops and they are on *terra firma*. The natural method for preventing motion sickness is to look at a point on the horizon, thus minimizing the motion exaggeration. On a large plane, stare at a distant cloud, or if you're stuck in a center seat look as far forward in the plane as possible. Reading tends to increase the symptoms. Avoid alcohol and greasy foods on bouncy trips. With repeated exposure to the same sort of motion, you may become adapted and experience less discomfort.

To medically prevent and treat *motion sickness* ("better living through chemistry"), a very useful medication in the Non-Rx Oral Medication Module is diphenhydramine 25 mg, taken 1 hour prior to departure and repeated every 6 hours as needed. This is not an indicated use for this medication and treatment or prevention of nausea will not be noted on the package. But it works, although drowsiness may be a problem for some (see page 221). Transderm Scope, a patch containing scopalamine, has been developed for prevention of motion sickness, but this requires a prescription. Each patch may be worn behind the ear for 3 days. It is fairly expensive, but very worthwhile if you are prone to this malady. There tends to be a higher frequency of side effects in elderly people with this medication, consisting of visual problems, confusion, and loss of temperature regulation. A valuable drug to prevent and treat motion sickness is Atarax 25 mg every 4 hours as needed from the Rx Oral/Topical Module, or Vistaril 25 mg IM every 4 hours as needed from the Rx Injectable Medication Module.

Diarrhea

Diarrhea is the expulsion of watery stool. This malady is usually self-limited, but can be a threat to life, depending upon its cause and extent. Diarrhea can be the result of bowel disorders such as diverticulitis or colitis, infectious diseases such as cholera, shigella, salmonella, and many other creatures borne in contaminated food or water, and rarely with appendicitis and gall bladder disease. The serious infectious disease malaria can have diarrhea as a presenting complaint. Obviously diagnosing the cause of diarrhea can be of importance both in regard to treating and in estimating the danger to the patient.

Diverticulitis is usually found in people over the age of 40 and is generally only a condition of the elderly. Diverticula are little pouches that form on the large intestine, or colon, from a weakness that develops over time in the muscles of its wall. These are of no trouble unless they become infected. Infection causes diarrhea, fever, and painful cramping. Pain is usually located along the left side of the abdomen. It tends to be at a constant location unlike many conditions with diarrhea where the pain migrates around. Appendicitis pain is in the right lower quadrant of the abdomen (see page 66). Treatment is with antibiotics such as the Levaquin 500 mg daily or Rocephin 500 mg given by injection twice daily.

Colitis and other inflammations of the bowel cause repeated bouts of diarrhea. At times a fever may be present. These cases are chronic, and like diverticulitis, the diagnosis must be made with barium enema x-ray or colonoscopy. If in doubt treat with antibiotics as indicated under diverticulitis. Both conditions require specific drugs for treatment, such as the steroids included with the Rx Oral/Topical and Injectable Modules, but unless the person has a prior history of these diseases, the use of such drugs in the wilderness is inappropriate.

Traveler's diarrhea is caused by infections, so prevention seems an appropriate priority. Prevention is effected by staying alert. Water sources must be known to be pure or treated as indicated on pages 83–87. Once dehydrated or freeze-dried food has been reconstituted, it should be stored as carefully as any fresh, unprocessed food. Be wary of fresh fruits and vegetables in developing countries. Peel all such items, or thoroughly rinse with purified water, or boil for 10 minutes minimum. It is almost impossible to peel anything but a banana without contaminating it, as a knife cutting through a contaminated peel will contaminate the inside. Often, in countries lacking refrigeration, fruits and vegetables are "freshened" on the way to the market by being sprinkled frequently with water from roadside drainage ditches. The use of human fertilizer makes this water very contaminated. This contamination is not eliminated by drying or wiping with a cloth. If the item being sold in the market is sold by weight, such as a melon, be careful! Some merchants inject roadside water into their product to increase its weight and value. Certain animal products are tainted in various parts of the world, particularly at specific times of the year. Know the flora and fauna that your expedition plans to utilize from local sources!

Diarrhea is diagnosed when an individual has 2 to 3 times the number of customary bowel movements for that individual. These stools can be either soft, meaning that they will take the shape of a container, or watery, meaning that they can be poured. By definition at least one associated symptom of fever, chills, abdominal cramps, nausea, or vomiting must be present. This will generally mean 4 unformed stools in a day, or 3 unformed stools in an 8 hour period when accompanied by at least one other symptom listed above.

The disease is generally self-limiting, lasting 2 to 3 days. As many as 75% of people will have abdominal pain and cramps, 50% will have nausea, and 25% will have vomiting and fever. An acute onset of watery diarrhea usually means that an enterotoxigenic *E. coli* is the cause, but shigellosis will also first present in this manner. Symptoms of bloody diarrhea or mucoid stools are frequently seen with invasive pathogens such as *Shigella, campylobacter,* or *Salmonella.* The presence of chronic diarrhea with malabsorption and gas indicates possible Giardia. Rotavirus disease starts with vomiting in 80% of cases.

In a study of U.S. students in Mexico, the cause of diarrhea was found to be: enterotoxigenic *E. coli* 40%; enteroadherent *E. coli* 5%; *Giardia lamblia* and *Entamoeba histolytica* 2%; rotavirus 10%; aeromonas 1%; *Shigella* 15%; *Salmonella* 7%; *campylobacter* 3%; and unknown 17%. Studies of traveler's diarrhea show different frequencies from the above in various other locations of the world, but the cause is always due to infection.

Various medications have been shown effective in prevention of traveler's diarrhea, but a 1985 consensus of experts discouraged their use due to cost, exposing people to drug side effects, possible development of resistant germs due to antibiotic overuse, and the normally benign course of the disease. Pepto-Bismol 2 ounces (4 tablespoons) or 2 tablets taken 4 times daily can prevent this problem. Ugh! There is about 8 aspirin tablets worth of salicylate in that quantity of Pepto-Bismol. Prevention with antibiotic is effective, although not usually indicated. The choice of antibiotic for either prevention or treatment depends on where in the world you are traveling. For prevention in Mexico, doxycycline 100 mg taken once daily should suffice. Elsewhere in the world, Levaquin 500 mg once daily would be a better choice.

Treating diarrhea with Pepto-Bismol requires 2 tablespoons every 30 minutes for 8 doses. As most diarrhea in developing countries is from bacterial causes, the use of antibiotics can be very effective. A single dose of the antibiotic Levaquin 500 mg can eliminate diarrhea instantly. Loperamide 2 mg, from the Non-Rx Oral Medication Module, may not be required if you have access to the Levaquin. A dose of loperamide may be given simultaneously with the Levaquin. When using the loperamide, give 2 tablets at once, followed by 1 tablet after each loose stool with a maximum adult dose of 8 tablets per day. One tablet of the pain medication Lorcet 10/650 can also stop diarrhea, but it would be best to use the loperamide and/or Levaquin if they are available.

Constipation

One of the popular wilderness medical texts has instructions on how to break up a fecal impaction digitally (i.e., using your finger to break up a hard stool stuck in the rectum). Don't let it get that far. In healthy young adults (especially teenagers), there may be a reluctance to defecate in the wilderness due to the unusual surrounding, lack of a toilet, and perhaps swarms of insects or freezing cold. It is the group leader's responsibility to make sure that a trip member does not fecal hoard, i.e., fail to defecate in a reasonable length of time. Certainly one should be concerned after 3 days of no bowel movements.

To prevent this problem, I always include a stewed fruit at breakfast on the expedition menu. The use of hot and cold food and water in the morning will frequently wake up the "gastric-colic reflex" and get things moving perfectly well. If the five-day mark is approaching, especially if the patient—and they have become a patient at about this point—is obviously uncomfortable, it may become necessary to use a laxative. From the medical kit (Non-Rx Oral Medication Module) give 1 bisacodyl laxative tablet 5 mg at bedtime. If that fails, the next morning take 2 of the tablets. Under winter conditions, when getting up in sub-zero weather might prove abominable, or under heavy insect conditions, take these tablets in the morning, rather than at night, to preclude this massive inconvenience occurring in the middle of the night. Any laxative will cause abdominal cramping, depending upon how strong it is. Expect this.

Hemorrhoids

Also called "piles," this painful swelling is a cluster of varicose veins around the rectum. External hemorrhoids are small, rounded purplish masses that enlarge when straining at stool. Unless a clot forms in them, they are soft and non-tender. When clots form, they can become very painful, actually excruciating. Hemorrhoids are the most common cause of rectal bleeding, with the blood also appearing on the toilet tissue. The condition can be very painful for about 5 days, after which the clots start to absorb, the pain decreases, and the mass regresses, leaving only small skin tags. Provide the patient with pain medication (non-Rx item) Percogesic 2 tablets every 4 hours. The application of heat is helpful during the acute phase. Heat a cloth in water and apply for 15 minutes 4 times a day if possible. Avoid constipation, as mentioned in that section. If you are carrying the Rx Oral/Topical Module, Topicort .25%

ointment will provide the anti-inflammation ability of a steroid and some local pain relief.

Hernia

The most common hernia in a male is the inguinal hernia, an out-pouching of the intestines through a weak area in the abdominal wall located above and on either side of the groin. It is through this area that the spermatic cord connects the testes to the back of the penis. A hernia can be produced while straining or lifting, even coughing or sneezing, when the bowel pushes along the spermatic cord. There will be a sharp pain at the location of the hernia and the patient will note a bulge. This bulge may disappear when he lies on his back and relaxes (i.e., the hernia has reduced). If the intestine in the hernia is squeezed by the ab-dominal wall to the point that the blood supply is cut off, the hernia is termed a "strangulated" hernia. This is a medical emergency, as the loop of gut in the hernia will die, turn gangrenous, and lead to a generalized peritonitis or abdominal infection (*peritonitis* is discussed under appen-dicitis). This condition is much worse than appendicitis and death will result if not treated surgically.

The hernia that fails to reduce or disappear when the victim relaxes in a recumbent position, is termed "incarcerated." While this may turn into an emergency, it is not one at that point. Most hernias caused by straining in adults will not strangulate. Further straining should be avoided. If lifting items is necessary, or coughing cannot be prevented, etc., the victim should protect himself from further tissue damage by pressing against the area with one hand, thus holding the hernia in re-duction. It can be a rather awkward way to carry a canoe.

Bladder Infection

The hallmarks of *bladder infection* (cystitis) are the urge to urinate fre-quently, burning upon urination, small amounts of urine being voided with each passage, and discomfort in the suprapubic region—the lowest area of the abdomen. Frequently the victim has fever with its attendant chills and muscle ache. In fact, people can become quite ill with a gen-eralized infection caused by numerous bacteria entering their blood-stream. At times the urine becomes cloudy and even bloody. Cloudy urine without the above symptoms does *not* mean an infection is present and is frequently normal. The infection can extend to the kidney, at which time the patient also has considerable flank pain, centered at the bottom edge of the ribs along the lateral aspect of the back on the involved side (often both sides). While bladder infections are more common in women than men, they are not an uncommon problem in either sex. One suffering from recurrent infections should be thoroughly evaluated by a physician prior to an extended wilderness trip.

There have been many drugs developed for treating infections of the genito-urinary system. The antibiotics recommended for the Rx medical kits all work excellently here. Doxycycline 100 mg taken 1 tablet twice daily is very effective. Levaquin 500 mg tablet once daily is ideal to use if the doxycycline seems ineffective. Generally 3 days is a sufficient length of time for treatment. Symptoms should disappear within 24 to 48 hours, or it may mean that the bacteria is resistant to the antibiotic and the other should be substituted.

For severe infections, with high fever that has not responded within 48 hours to oral antibiotic use, the injectable Rocephin 500 mg IM given twice daily in place of the oral antibiotic would be a superior choice.

Additional treatment should consist of drinking copious amounts of fluid, at least 8 quarts per day! At times this simple rinsing action may even cure a cystitis, but I wouldn't want to count on it. Use an antibiotic if it is available. Discomfort may be relieved by Percogesic from the non-Rx supplies, or one half a Lorcet 10/650 from the Rx Oral/Topical Module, but these are seldom required due to the rapid onset of relief following administration of the antibiotic. The Percogesic or ibuprofen may be needed to treat the fever that accompanies such problems prior to the start of the antibiotic and during the early the early stages of therapy.

Reproductive Organs

Venereal Diseases

Venereal infections are totally preventable by abstention; any other technique falls short of being foolproof. Most venereal infections cause symptoms in the male, but frequently do not in the female. Either may note increased discomfort with urination, the development of sores or unusual growths around the genitalia, and discharge from the portions of the anatomy used in sex (pharynx, penis, vagina, anus). Some venereal diseases can be very difficult to detect, such as syphilis, hepatitis B, and AIDS. Hepatitis B is rampant in many parts of the world with high carrier rates in local population groups. It can be prevented with a vaccine (see Appendix B). These are no vaccines against the other venereal diseases.

Gonorrhea is common and easy to detect in the male. The appearance of symptoms is from 2 to 8 days from time of contact and basically consists of a copious greenish-yellow discharge. The female will frequently not have symptoms. From the Rx kit provide doxycycline 100 mg twice daily for 15 days, to ensure adequate treatment of syphilis, which may have been caught at the same time.

Syphilis has an incubation period of 2 to 6 weeks before the characteristic sore appears. The development of a painless ulcer (0.25 to 0.5 inch or 0.6 to 1.2 cm in size), generally with enlarged, non-tender lymph nodes in the region, is a hallmark of this disease. A painful ulcer formation is more characteristic of herpes simplex. The lesion may not appear in a syphilis victim, making the early detection of this disease very difficult. A second stage consisting of a generalized skin rash (which usually does not itch, does not produce blisters, and frequently appears on the soles of the feet and palms of the hands) appears about 6 weeks after the lesions mentioned above. The third phase of the disease may develop in several years, during which nearly any organ system in the body may be affected. The overall study of syphilis is so complicated that a great medical instructor once said, "To know syphilis is to know medicine." Treatment of primary stage syphilis is 15 days of antibiotics, as mentioned above.

Development of a clear, scanty discharge in the male may be due to *chlamydia* or other nonspecific urethral infections. Symptoms appear 7 to 28 days after contact. Women may have no symptoms. Treat with doxycycline 100 mg twice daily for 15 days. Blood tests for syphilis should be performed before treatment and again in 3 months. 20% of victims with nonspecific urethritis will have a relapse, therefore adequate medical follow-up after the trip is essential.

Herpes lesions can respond to Denavir 1% cream applied frequently during the day until they disappear in 8 to 10 days. Famvir capsules 125 mg taken 3 times daily for 7 days are effective during the acute phase.

Upon returning home, members who may have experienced a sexual disease should be seen by their physician for serology tests for syphilis, hepatitis B tests, chlamydia smears, gonorrheal cultures, herpes simplex titers, and possibly HIV studies for AIDS. Lesions or growths should be examined as possible *molluscum contagiosum* and venereal warts should be treated.

Vaginal Discharge and Itching

Vaginal discharge and/or itching are frequently not indicators for venereal disease. The most common cause is a fungal or monilia infection. This condition is more common in conditions of high humidity or with the wearing of tight clothes such as pants or panty hose.

A typical monilia infection has a copious white discharge with curds like cottage cheese. From the Non-Rx Oral Module one can use the clotrimazole 1% cream. This formulation has been designed for foot and other skin fungal problems, but it will work vaginally as well. From the Rx Oral Medication Module use one Diflucan 150 mg tablet for treatment.

A frothy greenish-yellow, irritating discharge may be due to trichomonas infection. This can be spread by sexual encounters. The male infected with this organism generally has no symptoms, or a slight mucoid discharge early in the morning, noted before urinating. The treatment of choice is Flagyl (metronidazole) 250 mg capsule 3 times a day for 10 days, or 8 capsules given as one dose. This drug cannot be taken with alcohol. Sexual abstention is important until medication is finished and a cure is evident clinically. Generic Flagyl is frequently available in third world countries at pharmacies without a prescription.

A copious yellow-green discharge may indicate gonorrhea. Any irritating discharge that is not thick and white is best treated with the Levaquin 500 mg once daily. If sexual contact may have been the source of the problem, treat for 15 days to also kill any syphilis that may have been caught simultaneously. A douche of very dilute Hibiclens surgical scrub, or very dilute detergent solution, can be prepared and may be helpful. Very dilute is better than too strong. Frequent douching is not required, but it may be for a few days as required for comfort and hygiene.

Painful Testicle

If pain is severe, provide support by having the victim lie on the insulated ground with a cloth draped over both thighs, forming a sling or cradle on which the painful scrotum may rest. If ambulatory, provide support to prevent movement of the scrotum. Cold packs would help initially and providing adequate pain and nausea medication as available is certainly appropriate. Antibiotic is not required unless a fever results.

Spontaneous pain in the scrotum, with enlargement of a testicle, can be due to an infection of the testicle (orchitis) or more commonly to an infection of the sperm-collecting system called the epididymis (epididymitis). Treatment of choice would be to provide antibiotic such as the doxycycline 100 mg 1 tablet twice daily or Levaquin 500 mg once daily. Pain medication should be provided as necessary.

The problem may not be due to an infection at all. It is possible for the testicle to become twisted, due to a slight congenital defect, with severe pain resulting. This "testicular torsion," as it is called, is a surgical emergency. It can be almost impossible to distinguish from orchitis. In a suspected case of torsion it is helpful to try to reduce the torsion. Since the testicle always seems to rotate "inward," one need only rotate the affected testicle "outward." This will often result in immediate relief of the pain. If you cannot achieve this, or if you are dealing with an orchitis, no harm is done; but if it is a torsion, you have saved the testicle and the trip. A person with severe testicular pain should be evacuated as soon as possible as infection or torsion can result in sterility of the involved side. An unreduced testicular torsion can become gangrenous with life-threatening infection resulting.

Menstrual Problems

Menstrual flow is best contained in the wilderness with a vaginally inserted tampon, but be sure to have experience with the chosen product prior to heading backcountry. A resealable plastic bag should be carried if it is necessary to pack out discarded pads. Rolling several Nu-Gauze pads from the Topical Bandaging Module will substitute as an outer sanitary napkin if none is available. Menstrual cramping can generally be controlled with ibuprofen 200 mg 1 or 2 tablets every 4 to 6 hours from the Non-Rx Oral Medication Module. While this medication is used as an antiarthritic, its antiprostaglandin activities make it an ideal medication for the treatment of menstrual pain. From the Rx Oral/Topical Module, if necessary, one could use Lorcet 10/650 1 tablet every 6 hours as required.

Menorrhagia, either excessive flow or long period of flowage, should be evaluated by a physician to determine if there is an underlying pathology that could or should be corrected. If the problem is simply one of hormone imbalance, this can frequently be corrected with the use of birth control pills with higher amounts of estrogen and lower progestogen content. Consult a physician well in advance of the wilderness outing, so that these symptoms can be brought under control by the time of the expedition.

Spontaneous Abortion

Bleeding during pregnancy is not unusual—20 to 30% of women bleed or cramp during the first 20 weeks of their pregnancy. This is termed *threatened abortion* and is treated with bed rest, since this usually decreases the bleeding and cramping. 10 to 15% of pregnant women will go on to abort. As long as all products of the abortion pass—a "complete abortion"—the bleeding and pain stop and the uterus shrinks back to its normal size.

An incomplete abortion, the expulsion of only a portion of the fetus or the rupture of the membranes only, will often require a surgeon's care to perform a D&C. However, urgent evacuation is always mandatory. Watch for signs of sepsis, such as elevated temperature, and start antibiotic if possible. Give the Rocephin 1 gram IM, followed by 500 mg IM every 12 hours. The best oral antibiotic recommended for your kit would be the Levaquin 500 mg given daily. Give pain medication as necessary.

Ectopic Pregnancy

In an ectopic pregnancy, spotting and cramping usually begin shortly after the first missed period. If a pregnancy test is positive and the woman has severe lower abdominal pain lasting more than 24 hours, you probably have a surgical emergency on your hands. A rupture of the uterine tube usually occurs at 6 to 8 weeks of pregnancy, while a rupture of the cornual pregnancy occurs at 12 to 16 weeks. The rupture causes massive blood loss with a rapid onset of shock and death when it occurs.

While other causes of spotting during pregnancy are possible, you are in no position to handle any of them in the wilderness. Evacuate this woman urgently.

If a woman is having spotting, lower abdominal pain, and the pregnancy test is negative, you are in no position to bet her life that she is not pregnant. Ectopic pregnancies have lower blood levels of ß subunit HCG hormone to detect and the test may, therefore, be falsely negative.

Poisoning

Plant or Food Poisoning

The Pittsburgh Poison Control Center manages the vast majority of their poison plant ingestion victims by inducing vomiting with syrup of ipecac. One-half ounce (15 ml) of syrup of ipecac is given orally and two 8 oz (total 500 ml) glasses of water follow to enhance vomiting. This technique provides superior emptying compared to gastric lavage (stomach pumping) and can even cause the expulsion of particles in the upper portion of the small intestine. If no vomiting occurs, repeat the dose of ½ oz of syrup of ipecac in 20 minutes. If all fails, induce vomiting by gagging the throat with a finger or spoon. This latter technique may well be the only method available while in the bush.

Petroleum Products Poisoning

The danger from accidentally drinking various petroleum products—while siphoning from one container to another—is the possibility of accidentally inhaling or aspirating this liquid into the lungs. That will kill. The substances are not toxic enough in the GI tract to warrant the danger of inducing vomiting. Do not worry about swallowing several mouthfuls of any petroleum product. If the person vomits, there is nothing you can do about it, except position him so that there is less chance of aspiration into the lungs—sitting, bending forward is probably ideal. The more volatile the substance, the more the danger of aspiration. In other words, kerosene is less dangerous than Coleman fuel.

If organic phosphorous pesticides are dissolved in the fuel, you have a more complex problem. These substances are potentially toxic and must be removed. In the emergency room this would be accomplished by gastric lavage, or stomach pumping. In the bush, if you cannot evacuate the person within 12 hours, you will have to take a chance of inducing vomiting, with possible lethal aspiration—to eliminate the poison. Treat with ipecac or by inducing gagging as described under poison plant ingestion. After vomiting, administer a slurry of activated charcoal, if available. This helps bind unvomited toxins. Charcoal powder, to which you add water to form a slurry, is available at pharmacies. In the field you might consider tearing apart a charcoal water filter and crushing the charcoal granules. Or you can make the slurry from the blackened, partially burnt portions of logs from a campfire.

Ciguatera Poisoning

Ciguatera poisoning is caused by a toxin released by a small ocean organism called a dinoflagellate. As various species of fish eat this small plant they acquire the toxin. Larger fish that in turn prey on the smaller fish acquire larger and larger amounts of the toxin and thus result in more severe cases of ciguatera toxin poisoning in humans. Over 400 species of fish from the tropical reefs of Florida, the West Indies, and the Pacific have been implicated, but most often it has been barracuda, grouper, and amberjacks that are contaminated. No deep-sea fish such as tuna, dolphin, or wahoo have been found contaminated.

There is no way to detect contamination—no change in flavor, texture, or color of the fish flesh. Worse yet, no method of preserving, cooking, or treating fish can destroy this toxin. One must rely on local knowledge to avoid potentially polluted species.

Symptoms usually start with numbness and tingling of the lips and tongue, and then progress to dry mouth, abdominal cramping, vomiting and diarrhea that lasts 6 to 17 hours. Muscle and joint pain, muscle weakness, facial pain, and unusual sensory phenomena such as reversal of hot and cold sensations develop. Occasionally, low blood pressure, respiratory depression, and coma can result. Neurological symptoms are made worse by alcohol and exercise. Start rescue breathing if necessary (see page 19). From 1983 through 1992 508 cases were reported to the U.S. Centers for Disease Control and Prevention, mostly from Hawaii, with no deaths.

See also on *scromboid poisoning* and *paralytic shellfish poisoning.*

Scromboid Poisoning

The flesh of dark meat fish, such as tuna, mackerel, albacore, bonito, amberjack, and mahi-mahi (dolphin), contain large amounts of histadine. Improper storage after catching these fish allows bacterial enzymatic changes of this meat, releasing large amounts of histamine and other toxic by-products that are not destroyed by cooking.

Symptoms of scromboid poisoning include flushing, dizziness, headache, burning of the mouth and throat, nausea, vomiting, and diarrhea. Severe poisoning can cause significant respiratory distress. Diphenhydramine has been reported to cause an increase in symptoms at times, which is surprising since it is an excellent antihistamine. Cimetidine (Tagamet) from the Non-Rx Oral Medication Module has been shown to block the effects of scromboid poisoning. Give 4 200 mg tablets every

6 hours. While normally a prescription product used to control stomach acid formation, its mode of action is known as an H-2 histamine blocker. Other similar compounds in this class will have to be tested (Zantac, Pepcid, Axid), but if they are available they might be tried in an emergency.

Pufferfish Poisoning

Incorrectly prepared pufferfish (Fugu) contains tetrodotoxin, which can be lethal as it leads to respiratory failure and cardiac collapse. Symptoms may be slow in onset. Provide CPR as necessary (see page 19). More people are probably killed by ingesting poisonous marine creatures than are killed by any other form of encounter with them. There is certainly a tragedy when the predator becomes the victim, especially when it is us!

Paralytic Shellfish Poisoning

Mussels, clams, oysters, and scallops may ingest the poison saxitoxin from dinoflagellates known as the "red tide" from June to October along the New England and Pacific coasts. Numbness around the mouth may occur within 5 to 30 minutes after eating. Other symptoms are similar to ciguatera poisoning. These include gastrointestinal illness, loss of coordination, and paralysis progressing to complete respiratory paralysis with 12 hours in 8% of cases. No specific treatments or antidotes are available, but purging of stomach contents should be encouraged. Artificial support of respirations is potentially life-saving.

Managing Diabetes

Diabetic children or adults can have an active outdoor life, but learning to control their diabetes must first be worked on with their physicians. The increased caloric requirement of wilderness exercise may range above an extra 2,000 calories per day, yet insulin dosage requirements may drop as much as 50%. The diabetic as well as the trip partners must be able to identify the signs of low blood sugar (hypoglycemia)—staggering gait, slurred speech, moist skin, clumsy movements—and know the proper treatment, i.e. oral carbohydrates, or sugar candies and, if the patient becomes unconscious, the use of injectable glucagon. Urine of diabetic outdoor travelers should be tested twice daily to confirm control of sugar. This testing should preclude a gradual accumulation of too much blood sugar, which can result in unconsciousness in its far advanced stage. This gradual accumulation would have resulted in massive sugar spill in the urine, and finally the spill of ketone bodies, providing the patient ample opportunity to increase insulin dosage to prevent hyperglycemia (too high a blood sugar level).

Storage of insulin in the wilderness, where it forgoes recommended refrigeration, is not a major problem so long as the supply is fresh and direct sunlight and excessive heat is avoided. Syringes, alcohol prep pads, Keto-diastix urine test strips, insulin, and glucagon are light additions to the wilderness medical kit.

Water and Waste

Oral Fluid Replacement Therapy

Replacement of fluid loss is required for three different circumstances: diarrhea, heat stress sweat formation, and insensible moisture loss from breathing and skin respiration (yes, skin must breathe also). The ideal fluid replacement for each of these losses differs in electrolyte and sugar content. In general, diarrhea replacement fluids should not have a greater sugar content than 2.5% as a higher concentration might cause additional diarrhea. (A higher sugar concentration is not a problem in a person who is not ill.) Sweat replacement solutions should not have a sugar concentration greater than 8.5%, this slows the emptying of the fluid from the stomach. The uptake of water by the body is decreased as this occurs in the intestines and not the stomach. The ideal electrolyte composition for these circumstances also differs dramatically.

Profound diarrhea from any source may cause severe dehydration and electrolyte imbalance. The nonvomiting patient must receive adequate fluid replacement, equaling his stool loss plus about 2 liters per day. An adult can replace these losses by drinking enough plain water. A child, or less healthy adult, will require electrolyte replacement in addition to the water. The Centers for Disease Control and Prevention recommends the oral replacement cocktails for fluid losses caused by profound diarrhea, seen in Table 2–7.

Drink alternately from each glass. Supplement with carbonated beverages or water and tea made with boiled or carbonated water as desired. Avoid solid foods and milk until recovery.

Throughout the world UNICEF and WHO distribute an electrolyte replacement product called Oralyte. It must be reconstituted with ade-

Table
2-7

Oral Replacement Cocktails

Prepare two separate glasses of the following:

Glass 1)   Orange, apple or other fruit juice
(rich in potassium)......................8 ounces
Honey or corn syrup (glucose necessary
for absorption of essential salts).........½ tsp
Salt, table (rich in sodium and chloride)..1 pinch

Glass 2)   Water (carbonated or boiled)..............8 ounces
Soda, baking (sodium bicarbonate)..........¼ tsp

quately purified water. These packets can be hard to obtain and expensive in the United States, but a source is listed in the Web site.

If the patient is maintaining fluid balance with an effective oral rehydration therapy, such as with the packets as indicated above, the additional glass of carbonated or bicarbonate water is not necessary. Other products that are considered safe for rehydration due to diarrheal losses are Naturalyte, Pedialyte, Infalyte, and Pediatric. Gatorade is too high in carbohydrate and too low in sodium, potassium, and base to be considered a safe substitute, even with modification.

Water Purification

Water can be purified adequately for drinking by mechanical, physical, and chemical means.

The clearest water possible should be chosen or attempts made to clarify the water prior to starting any disinfectant process. Water with high particulate count, with clay or organic debris, allows high bacterial counts and tends to be more heavily contaminated. In preparing potable, or drinkable, water we are attempting to lower the germ counts to the point that the body can defend itself against the remaining numbers. We are not trying to produce sterile water, that would generally be impractical.

The use of chlorine-based systems has been effectively used by municipal water supply systems for years. There are two forms of chlorine readily available to the outdoors traveler. One is liquid chlorine laundry bleach and the other is Halazone tablets.

Laundry bleach that is 4 to 6 percent sodium hypochlorite can make clear water safe to drink if 2 drops are added to 1 quart of water. Avoid brands of bleach that contain soap or surfactant. This water must be mixed thoroughly and let stand for 30 minutes before drinking. The resulting blend should have a slight chlorine odor. If not, the original laundry bleach may have lost some of its strength and you should repeat the dose and let stand an additional 15 minutes prior to drinking.

Halazone tablets from Abbott Laboratories are also effective. They are actually quite stable with a shelf-life of 5 years, even when exposed to temperatures over 100° F (38° C) occasionally. Recent articles in outdoor literature have stated that Halazone has a short shelf-life and that it loses 75% of its activity when exposed to air for two days. Abbott Labs refutes this and has proven the efficacy of use for Halazone sufficiently to receive FDA approval. A clue to the stability of the tablets is that they turn yellow and have an objectionable odor when they decompose. Check for this before use. Five tablets should be added to a quart of clear water for adequate chlorination.

Chlorine-based systems are very effective against virus and bacteria. They work best in neutral or slightly acid waters. As the active form of the chlorine, namely, hypochlorous acid (HCLO), readily reacts with nitrogen containing–compounds such as ammonia; high levels of organic debris decrease its effectiveness. The amount of chlorine bleach or Halazone added must be increased if the water is alkaline or contaminated with organic debris.

Iodine is a fairly effective agent against protozoan contamination such as *Giardia lamblia* and *Entamoeba hystolytica,* which tend to be resistant to chlorine. Further, iodine is not as reactive to ammonia or other organic debris, thus working better in cloudy water. It is relatively ineffective against *Cryptosporidium,* which must be destroyed by either filtration or heat (see page 86). Tincture of iodine, as found in the home medicine chest, may be used as the source of the iodine. Using the commonly available 2% solution, 5 drops should be added to clear water or 10 drops to cloudy water, and the resultant mix should be allowed to stand 30 minutes prior to drinking.

The Armed Forces were responsible for developing a solid tablet that provided a source of iodine. Tetraglycine hydroperiodide is available as Globaline or Potable Aqua, or as Army surplus water purification tablets. An elemental iodine concentration of 3 to 5 ppm (part per million) is necessary to kill amoeba and their cysts, algae, bacteria and their spores, and enterovirus. Two tablets of Potable Aqua will provide 16 ppm iodine concentration per quart. If the water is clear, a 10 minute wait is required; for cloudy water wait 20 minutes before consuming. At near freezing temperatures, wait a full 30 minutes before drinking.

Crystals of iodine can also be used to prepare a saturated iodine water solution for use in disinfecting drinking water. Four to eight grams of USP grade iodine crystals can be placed in a 1 ounce glass bottle. Water added to this bottle will dissolve an amount of iodine based on its temperature. It is this saturated iodine water solution that is then added to the quart of water. The amount added to produce a final concentration of 4 ppm will vary according to temperature, as indicated in Table 2–8.

Iodine Concentrations for Water Disinfections

Table 2-8

TEMPERATURE	VOLUME	CAPFULS
37° F (3° C)	20.0cc	8
68° F (20° C)	13.0cc	5+
77° F (25° C)	12.5cc	5
104° F (40° C)	10.0cc	4

{FN}*Assuming 2.5 cc capacity for a standard 1 ounce glass bottle cap

This water should be stored for 15 minutes before drinking. If the water is turbid, or otherwise contaminated, the amounts of saturated iodine solution indicated above should be double and the resultant water stored 20 minutes before using. This product is now commercially available as PolarPure through many outdoor stores and catalog houses.

Mechanical filtration methods are also useful in preparing drinking water. They normally consist of a screen with sizes down to 6 microns in size which are useful in removing tapeworm eggs (25 microns) or *Giardia lamblia* (7 to 15 microns). These screens enclose an activated charcoal filter element, which removes many disagreeable tastes. As most bacteria have a diameter smaller that 1 micron, bacteria and the even smaller viral species are not removed by filtration using these units. For water to be safe after using one of these devices it must be pre-treated with chlorine or iodine exactly as indicated above prior to passage through the device. While these filters remove clay and organic debris, they will plug easily if the water is very turbid. A concern with the charcoal filter usage is that the filters may become contaminated with bacteria when they are used the next time. Pre-treating the water helps prevent this. I have frequently used a charcoal filter system to ensure safe, good tasting water after chemical treatment.

Another filtration method is perhaps one of the oldest, namely filtering through unglazed ceramic material. This was done in large crocks, a slow filtration method popular in tropical countries many years ago. A modern version of this old system is the development of a pressurized pump method. Made in Switzerland, the Katadyn Pocket Filter has a ceramic core enclosed in a tough plastic housing, fitted with an aluminum pump. The built-in pump forces water through the ceramic filter at a rate of approximately three-quarters of a quart per minute. Turbid water will plug the filter, but a brush is provided to easily restore full flow rates. This filter has a .2 micron size, which eliminates all bacteria and larger pathogens. Pre-treating of the water is not required. There is evidence that viral particles are also killed by this unit as the ceramic material is silver-impregnated, which appears to denature viruses as they pass through the filter. This possibility is being evaluated by the FDA at this time. I have worked with many groups using this device and they have had many favorable comments. These units are not cheap, costing about $240.00 retail. They weigh 23 ounces. There are several less expensive ceramic units now available, but be sure to pre-treat the water chemically when using these systems, as they may be ineffective against viral disease without the silver impregnation.

Another method of water purification has been with us a long time, namely using our old friend fire. Bringing water to a boil will effectively kill pathogens and make water safe to drink. One reads variously to boil water 5, 10, even 20 minutes. But simply bringing the water temperature to 150° F (65.5° C) is adequate to kill the pathogens discussed above, and all others besides. At high altitude the boiling point of water is reduced. For example, at 25,000 feet the boiling point of water is 185° F (85° C).

Bringing water to a boil is the minimal safe time for preparation. At times fuel or water may be in short supply and this minimal time must be used. It will never be necessary to boil water longer than 5 minutes and the shortest time mentioned (just bringing the water to a boil) will

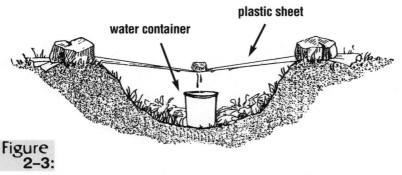

water container

plastic sheet

Figure
2-3:

Solar still condensing drinkable water from vegetation or contaminated sources. A solar still is very slow and produces minimal amounts of water.

suffice for a safe drinking water. This water will not be sterile, but it will be safe to drink.

Water may be obtained by squeezing any fresh water fish and some plants. Never drink urine or sea water, as the high solute content of these liquids will only dehydrate you more and make the problem worse. A solar still can be prepared for reprocessing urine, water from debris, or any moist material, as indicated in Figure 2–3. In water-poor areas, catching rain water may be an essential part of routine survival. Be careful of melting ice; treat all ice melt water as indicated above. There is a very strong chance of contamination of ice deposits.

Human Waste Disposal

This is not only a matter of esthetics but of primary preventative medicine. Improper waste disposal on the wagon trains heading west in the 1840s to 1850s caused vast epidemics of cholera in the trains that followed. Unbelievable numbers of people were killed. Even in our wilderness areas, it is widely acknowledged that the cleanest looking streams should be suspected of human contamination. Most official campsites in the national park system have toilets. These should always be used. Otherwise human defecation should be buried at least 200 feet (60 meters) from a lake shore or stream. Waste should be buried in a shallow pit as this promotes rapid decomposition. Disinfecting waste by adding undiluted bleach or solid bleach powder is a viable alternative. In very dry and seldom traveled areas, using the smear technique to dispose of feces is advocated. In some ecosystems all solid waste, including feces, must be carried out. General guidelines are available for different ecosystems and various levels of human usage.

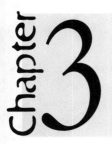

Chapter 3

Soft Tissue Care and Trauma Management

The Bleeding Wound

The first aid approach to a bleeding wound is to stop the bleeding, treat for shock, and transport the victim (with appropriate assessments) for definitive care. In remote areas it will frequently be very appropriate for the party to provide its own definitive care.

Stop the Bleeding

Wound care, whether in the wilderness or not, can be broken into chronological phases. The first phase consists of *saving the victim's life*—by stopping the bleeding and treating for shock. Even if the victim is not bleeding, you will want to treat for shock. Shock has many medical definitions, but bottom line, it amounts to an inadequate oxygenated blood supply getting to the brain. Lie the patient down, elevate feet above the head, and provide protection from the environment—from both the ground and the atmosphere. Grab anything that you can find for this at first—use jackets, pack frames, unrolled tents, whatever. Eventually you will be able to pitch a tent, put up a rain fly or sun shield, and prepare materials for further wound care. See also *shock, page 16.*

Direct pressure is the best method of stopping bleeding. In fact pressure alone can stop bleeding from amputated limbs! When the accident first occurs, you may even have to use your bare hand to stem the flow of blood. Ideally, you will have something to protect you from direct contact with blood and to protect the wound from your dirty hand. The best item to carry would be a pair of nitrile gloves. They can withstand long term storage as well as heat and cold better than latex gloves. Bottom line, grab a piece of cloth (bandanna, clothing article) or other barrier substance (plastic food wrapper) and press.

If direct pressure does not stop the bleeding, you may have to resort to the use of a tourniquet. Continue applying direct pressure while the tourniquet is on to facilitate the clotting process. Remove the tourniquet every 5 minutes, continuing to apply direct pressure, to see if adequate bleeding control can be obtained with the direct pressure alone. Repeat this as often as necessary. Sometimes bleeding control with direct pressure may require hours of direct pressure, but this is unusual. It is important that the tourniquet be only applied in 5 minute increments as this minimizes the chance for clots to form in the veins and ensures an adequate oxygen supply to tissues beyond the tourniquet site. Furthermore, an arterial tourniquet is extremely uncomfortable and can only be tolerated for more than 5 minutes by an unconscious person.

An alternate procedure to tourniquet use is to plunge two fingers into the bleeding wound. This always stops bleeding and works anywhere on the body. Use your index and middle finger held together. This is the technique used over and over again during surgery when something cuts loose and blood wells up in the surgical field.

A third technique is an internal pressure packing using a moist piece of sterile or clean cloth. Wet the cloth with sterile or at least drinkable water, wringing it out until it's practically dry. Then stuff this cloth into the wound firmly, continuing to pack more cloth into the wound until the bleeding is stopped by the tamponad, or compression. If bleeding continues do not remove the material, but firmly stuff in more. This dressing is covered with a dry clean cloth. It should be replaced in 24 hours.

With the blood stopped, even with your hand, and the victim on the ground in the shock treatment position, the actual emergency is over. Her life is safe. And you have bought time to gather together various items you need to perform the definitive job of caring for this wound. You have also treated for psychogenic shock—the shock of "fear." Obviously someone knows what to do: she has taken charge, she has stopped the bleeding, she is giving orders to gather materials together.

In the first aid management of this wound, the next step is simply bandaging and then transporting the victim to professional medical care. For those isolated in the wilderness, who must provide long-term care for wounds, further management will go through several more phases: cleaning, closing, dressing, and treating the possible complications of infection.

Clean the Wound

Adequate cleansing is the most important aspect of wound management. Especially when in an isolated or survival situation, the prevention of infection is of critical importance and can only be assured by aggressive irrigation techniques.

There is an adage in nature: "The solution to pollution is dilution." In wound care this means copious irrigation. The whole purpose of scrubbing a wound is to reduce the total number of potentially harmful bacteria. We won't get' em all out, but if the total number is sufficiently small, the body's own defense mechanisms can take over and finish the job for us.

To best provide water for irrigation, prepare sterile water. This can be done by boiling the water for 5 minutes. Lacking the ability to do this,

Figure 3-1:   The irrigating bulb syringe

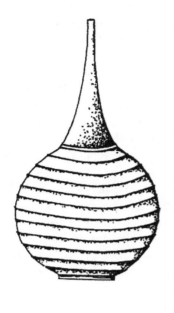

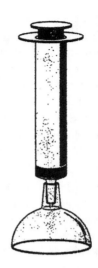

Figure 3-2:   The Zerowet Splashield attached to a syringe

try to use water that is fit for drinking (see page 83 for techniques of water purification). In a pinch, clean water from a stream or lake can be used as long as you are not downstream from the sewage pipe of a third world village or a bloated, rotting moose.

To provide adequate force to the irrigation stream, there are two items of potential importance. One is the bulb syringe (see Figure 3–1). The 1 oz model is adequate for most wilderness wounds. The other approach is to use a syringe (10 ml to 35 ml size) with a new device attached called a Zerowet Splashield (see Figure 3–2). With either technique one can increase the velocity of the water to aid in dislodging debris and those all important germs.

Forceful water irrigation is the mainstay of wound cleaning. The use of a "bota" bag, a squeezable plastic water cube, or simply a zip-locked baggy with a small hole poked in it to bring a stream of water to the wound is very helpful, but it really isn't adequate to provide the irrigation force required. Adding surgical scrub solution to the irrigation water is a good step but does not make up for the lack of forceful irrigation needed. Adding mechanical abrasion can be helpful and may be the only hope of adequate wound cleansing. Several products can be particularly useful for this technique. The most effective is Hibiclens surgical scrub. Another is povidone–iodine (Betadine) diluted to a 1% solution (the stock solution is 10%). Another approach is to use very dilute soap solution. Err on the side of making the soap solution too weak, because strong soap solutions can damage healthy tissue. Make the solution weak enough that you could drink it without purging yourself.

Many cleaning techniques and compounds *should not be used:* Tincture of iodine, mercurochrome, or alcohol are very harsh; hydrogen peroxide destroys good flesh as well as germs. Red–hot branding irons and pouring gun powder into a wound and lighting it, while effective in killing germs and among Rambo's favorite techniques, also destroy good tissue.

When stuck with a weak irrigation stream, perhaps only being able to pour water into the wound from a container, the mechanical abrasion technique saves the day. Besides irrigation, a technique of cleaning used by physicians in the operating room is called *debridement*. This amounts to cutting away destroyed tissue. Of course, there is no way a person can do this in the bush—especially with inadequate lighting, equipment, and training. But we *can* safely approximate it by vigorously rubbing the area with a piece of sterile gauze or clean cloth. The rigorous scrubbing action will remove blood clot, torn bits of tissue, pieces of foreign bodies—all items that generally result in higher bacteria counts or foci for bacterial growth. This scrubbing process has to be accomplished quickly—it is painful and the victim will not tolerate it for long. Have everything ready: clean, dry dressing to apply afterward; the water supply; an instrument to spread the wound open (a pair of tweezers or the needle holder are ideal); and sterile gauze to use for scrubbing this wound.

To sterilize cloth and any instruments, boil for 5 minutes, if necessary in the water you are preparing to use for irrigation. While having adequate sterile dressings would be ideal, you may find yourself slicing and dicing your wool shirt or Polarguard jacket into bandaging material. A rough cloth works better at wound cleaning than a smooth cloth, such as cotton.

Once everything is ready, and assistance is at hand (perhaps someone to squirt the jet of water into the wound and another to assist shooing the black flies away or comforting the victim), go to it! If this job is performed well, the final outcome will be great. This part of wound care is far more important than wound closure technique. It will be messy. And it will hurt. But spread the wound apart, blast that water in there the best you can, and scrub briskly with the gauze pad. *This whole process will have to be completed in 20 to 30 seconds.* In the operating room, or under local anesthesia in the emergency room, we might take 15 minutes or longer. You won't be able to take that much time, but you must be thorough and vigorous. Generally you should use at least 1 cup of water for a very small wound and 1 quart (1 liter) for most wounds. When in doubt, you must do more—if the patient can tolerate it within reason.

Once the irrigation is completed, the wound will bleed vigorously again, since the blood clots have been knocked off during the cleansing process. Apply a sterile dressing and use direct pressure as long as necessary to stop bleeding. Five to ten minutes usually suffice, but if an hour or more is required, keep at it or use the pressure dressing technique described above. If you fail to adequately clean a wound, the resulting infection could cost the patient his life. It would simply be a slower and more painful death than bleeding to death.

Antibiotic Guidelines

It is always tempting to place a person on antibiotics after a laceration, but I would advise against doing this unless the wound was from an animal or human bite (pages 110–11), the wound occurred in contaminated water, or there was an open fracture (page 127). Bacteria are jealous creatures and do not like to share their food source with other species. If an infection develops, it will generally be a pure culture, the other species originally contaminating the wound having been killed off by the body defense mechanisms and the winning bacterium. If the patient is on an antibiotic from the beginning, the winning bacterium is guaranteed to resist your medication. If no antibiotic is used initially, there is hope that the emergent bacterium will be sensitive to the antibiotic that you are about to employ.

If it is necessary to start a prophylactic antibiotic, from the Rx Oral/Topical Medication Module, use Levaquin 500 mg once daily. Use this for 3 days. In case of infection, see page 114.

Wound Closure Techniques

With direct pressure still applied, dry around the wound. We are ready to now enter the wound closure phase of wound care. Perhaps more worry and concern exists about this phase of wound care than the others, but it is really the easiest—and much less important than the first two phases just discussed.

Tape Closure Techniques

If the laceration can be held together with tape, by all means use tape as the definitive treatment. Butterfly bandages are universally available, and generally work very well. The commercial butterflies are superior to homemade in that they are packaged sterile with a no-stick center portion. They can be made in the field by cutting and folding the center edges in to cover the adhesive in the very center of short tape strips, thus avoiding adhesive contact with the wound. Of course such homemade strips will not be sterile, but in general they will be very adequate.

The best tape closure system today is the Spyroflex wound dressing. It is very adherent, very conformable to body contours, can be cut into ideal shapes, and provides a definitive "smart" dressing that can be left in place until the wound heals (see page 215). No outer bandage covering is required with Spyroflex, so carrying it allows you to reduce the amount of bandage material in your medical kit considerably.

The Spyroflex is usually adequate to secure even stretched stressed wound sites and it makes a good direct cover over missing tissue areas. However, if you use tape strips of any type, there may be times when they cannot hold a wound closed and the wound will have to be stapled or sutured (stitched).

Stapling

A fast, strong method of holding skin edges together is with the use of stainless steel staples. A special disposable device will contain a certain number of sterile staples that rapidly staple the wound edges while pinching the wound together. This obviously stings while being used, but the pain is brief and the wound is secure. A very useful device is the Precise Five-Shot Skin Stapler by 3–M Corp., which obviously contains 5 staples. A special disposable staple remover is very handy for taking staples out virtually painlessly. The skin stapler and staple remover are non-prescription and shown in Figure 3–3. They come packaged in sterile, water-proof containers.

Suturing

Suture (stitching) material is available in many forms and with many types of needles. For the expedition medical kit, I would recommend

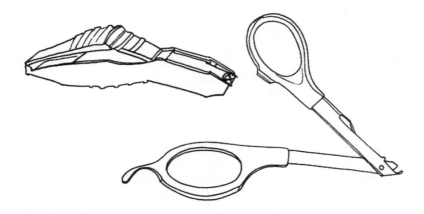

Figure
3-3:
The Precise Five-Shot Skin Stapler and its companion staple extraction device.

using 3–0 nylon suture with a curved pre-attached needle, shown in Figure 3–4. This comes in a sterile packet ready for use. It will be necessary to use a needle holder to properly hold this suture. The needle holder looks like a pair of scissors, but it has a flat surface with grooves that grab the needle and a lock device that holds the needle firmly. It is held as illustrated to steady the hand. All fly-tying stores sell needle holders.

Apply pressure in the direction of the needle, namely twist your wrist

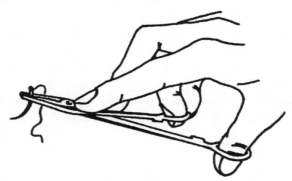

Figure
3-4:
Grasping the needleholder; this technique decreases hand tremor

is such a manner that the needle will pass directly into the skin and cleanly penetrate, following through with the motion to allow the needle to curve through the subcutaneous tissue and sweep upward and through the skin on the other side of the wound; see Figure 3–5.

Figure 3–5:

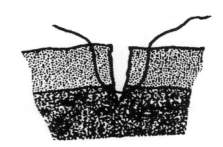

Proper placement of suture, showing passage of the suture material at an equal depth on both sides of the cut

Depth of Sutures

Suture through the skin surface only and avoid important structures underneath. If tendon or nerve damage has occurred, irrigate the wound thoroughly as described above and repair the skin with either tape or sutures as necessary. The tendon, etc., can be repaired by a surgeon upon return to the outside—weeks later if necessary.

It is important to have the needle enter both sides of the wound at the same depth or the wound will not pull together evenly and there will be a pucker if the needle took a deep bite on one side and a shallow bite on the other; see Figure 3–6.

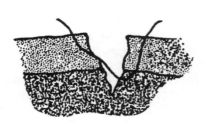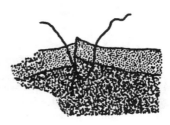

Figure 3–6:

Improper placement of suture, showing that different depths of penetration result in tissue puckering

A square knot is tied with the use of the needle holder in a very easy manner, as in Figure 3–7. Frankly, a knot tied in any fashion will do perfectly well.

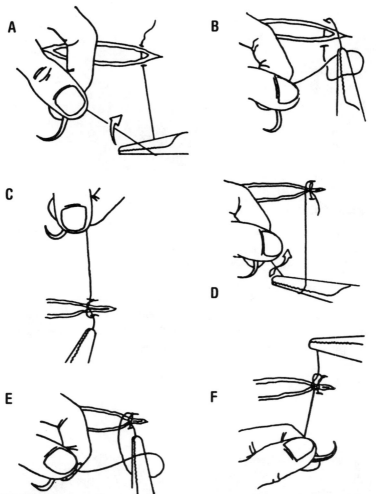

Figure 3–7: How to tie a square knot: (A) Loop the suture around the needle holder once, using the long end of the thread. (B and C) Grasp the short end and pull the wound together. (D and E) Loop the long end around the needle holder again the opposite way. This will form a square knot. Repeat this process a third time in the original direction to ensure a firm knot. Do not pull too tightly as this will pucker the skin; just an approximation is required.

Spacing of Staples and Sutures

These stitches should not be placed too closely together. Usually, on the limbs and body 4 stitches per inch will suffice. On the face, however, use 6 per inch. Here it is best to use 5-0 nylon, as it will minimize scar formation from the needle and suture. I use a 6-0 suture on the face, but it is considerably more difficult to use than the 5-0. These stitches can be combined with tape strips or butterfly bandages to help hold the wound together and to cut down on the number of stitches required. Once they are in, leave stitches in the limbs for 10 days, in the trunk and scalp for 7 days, and in the face for 4 days. A wound that tends to break open due to tension, such as over the knee, can be stabilized by splinting the joint so that it cannot move while the wound is healing.

Special Considerations

Shaving the Wound Area

It has been found that shaving an area increases the chance of wound infection. Scalp lacerations are hard to suture when unshaven due to the matting of hair with blood and accidental incorporation of hair into the wound. However, catching hair in the wound is not detrimental. Just pull it loose from the wound with a pair of forceps or tweezers when you are through suturing.

Bleeding from Suture or Staple Use

Anywhere on the body you will note that entrance and exit points of the needle puncture will bleed quite freely. A little pressure always stops the bleeding—it is not necessary to delay your sewing to even worry about it. Just complete your stitching of the wound, then apply pressure until the bleeding from the needle punctures stops, cleanse the skin when you are done to remove dried blood, and dress the wound.

Scalp Wounds

Scalp wounds bleed excessively—expect this. Spurting blood vessels can be clamped with the needle holder and tied off with a piece of the 3–0 gut suture in the surgical kit of the Topical Bandaging Module. To tie, simply place a knot in the flesh to fall beneath the tip of the needle holder. Someone may have to remove the needle holder while you are cinching the first loop of the knot. Or you may simply suture the scalp wound closed and apply pressure between each suture to minimize intra-operative bleeding. Apply firm direct pressure after suturing to minimize hematoma (blood pocket formation) from bleeding within the wound.

I have read many times that a scalp laceration can be closed by tying the hair on either side into a knot, thus holding the wound together. I have sutured a lot of scalp lacerations and I doubt this technique would work very well. A scalp laceration bleeds so profusely, blood is so sticky and slippery at the same time, and the hair would have to be long enough and of the right texture. See the discussion on *head injuries* on page 128.

Eyebrow and Lip Closure

If sewing an eyebrow or the vermilion border of the lip, approximate the edges first with a suture before sewing the ends or other portion of the laceration. Never shave an eyebrow. Use the 5-0 nylon suture on the face and remove these sutures in 4 days, replacing them with strips of tape at that time.

Mouth and Tongue Lacerations

When sewing the inside of the mouth, use the 3–0 gut suture. These sutures tend to unwind very easily, especially if the patient cannot resist touching them with his tongue. When making the knot, tie it over and over. As the mouth heals rapidly, if the sutures come out within a day, the laceration has generally stopped bleeding and may heal without further help. These mouth sutures will generally dissolve on their own, but remaining ones can be removed within 4 days.

Lacerations on the tongue can almost always be left alone. The wound may appear ugly for a few days, but within a week or two there will be remarkable healing. Infections in the tongue or mouth from cuts are very rare. If the edge of a tongue is badly lacerated, so that the tongue is cut one quarter of the way across or more, sewing the edge together is warranted. Use the 3–0 gut suture.

Control of Pain

For anesthesia you will require a prescription to obtain injectable lidocaine 1% and a syringe with needle. Inject through the wound, just under the skin on both sides of the cut. Cleansing and suturing soon

after a cut may help minimize the pain, due to tissue "shock" in the immediate posttrauma period. Ice applied to the wound area can help
numb the pain, but local topical anesthetic agents are of no help in pain
control. Two Percogesic or 1 Lorcet 10/650 given about 1 hour prior to
surgery, may help minimize pain.

Dressings

Most sutured lacerations will leak a little blood during the first 24
hours. The ideal covering would be the Spyroflex wound dressings as
mentioned on page 95. Any blood or serum drainage is easily absorbed
by this dressing. Leave it on for 10 days, until the wound is fully healed.
Increased pain, or apparent swelling is a reason to remove the dressing to
check for signs of infection (see page 114). The dressing should be removed, and replaced, when it is time to remove staples or sutures as indicated above. When used as a wound closure system by itself, it is not
necessary to remove this dressing as it facilitates more rapid healing and
provides protection from the environment while in place.

Alternative dressings in the Topical Bandaging Module are the Nu-
Gauze pads, the Tegoderm and the Spenco 2nd Skin dressings. An initial
covering that can soak up leaking wounds is the Nu-Gauze pads. After
the wound becomes dry, the Tegoderm dressing will keep the sutures
visible and the wound protected even if it must get submersed in water.
Wounds that continue to leak considerable serum and/or blood should
be covered by Spenco 2nd Skin and managed as discussed on page 216.

Other Types of Wounds

Abrasions

An abrasion is the loss of surface skin due to a scraping injury. The
best treatment is cleansing with Hibiclens surgical scrub, application of
triple antibiotic ointment, and the use of Spyroflex, all components of
the Topical Bandaging Module. This type of wound leaks profusely, but
the above bandaging allows rapid healing, excellent protection, and considerable pain relief. Avoid the use of alcohol on these wounds as it
tends to damage the tissue, to say nothing of causing excessive pain.
Lacking first aid supplies, cleanse gently with mild detergent and protect
from dirt, bugs, etc., the best that you can. Tetanus immunization should
be within 10 years.

A significant question on the mind of the victim and the medic is how aggressively should ground-in cinder and dirt be removed from a road rash. Having raced bicycles for several years on a cinder track (the Indiana University Little 500), I have had personal experience with this—which perhaps clouds my perspective. Before I raced, I aggressively cleaned these wounds with a wire brush. During my racing years my approach changed to simply coating the wound with a layer of the antibiotic ointment and allowing the resultant scab formation to lift the cinders out of the wound when it fell off. A recent publication has shown that antibiotic salve, if applied within 3 hours of a surface wound, significantly decreases wound infection in animal studies. I have not experienced problems with cinder tattoos or wound infection using gentle scrub with soft cloth—Hibiclens surgical scrub—removal of deeply imbedded debris carefully with tweezers, and a liberal coating of triple antibiotic ointment, reapplied daily or as necessary until the wound heals. I like to avoid a bandage, leaving the wound open to the air, or using the Spyroflex, when a covering is required, over the ointment.

Puncture Wound

Briefly allow a puncture wound to bleed, thus hoping to effect some irrigation of bacteria from the wound. Apply suction with the Sawyer Extractor (venom suction device) immediately and continue the vacuum for 10 minutes. Cleanse the wound area with surgical scrub or soapy water and apply triple antibiotic ointment to the surrounding skin surface. Do not tape shut, but rather start warm compress applications for 20 minutes, every 2 hours for the next 1 to 2 days, or until it is apparent that no sub-surface infection has started. These soaks should be as warm as the patient can tolerate without danger of burning the skin. Larger pieces of cloth work best as compresses, such as undershirts, as they hold the heat longer. Infection can be prevented, or treated, with antibiotics as described in the section on cellulitis, page 116. Dressing should be with a clean cloth. If sterile items are in short supply they need not be used on this type of wound. Tetanus immunization should be current (see Appendix B).

Splinter Removal

Prepare the wound with Hibiclens surgical scrub or other solution that does not discolor the skin. Minute splinters are hard enough to see. If the splinter is shallow, or the point buried, use a sharp blade to tease

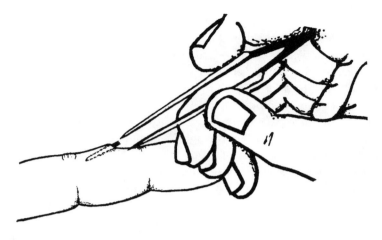

**Figure
3-8:**

**Hold tweezers parallel to the skin surface and grasp only
after obtaining adequate exposure of the splinter.**

the tissue over the splinter to remove this top layer. The splinter can
then be pried out better.

It is best to be aggressive in removing this top layer and obtaining a
substantial bite on the splinter with the tweezers, rather than nibbling
off the end when making futile attempts to remove with inadequate exposure. When using tweezers, grasp the instrument between the thumb
and forefinger, resting the instrument on the middle finger and further
resting the entire hand against the victim's skin, if necessary, to prevent
tremor. Approach the splinter from the side, if exposed, grasping it as
low as possible; see Figure 3-8. Apply triple antibiotic afterwards.

Tetanus immunization should be current. If the wound was dirty,
scrub afterwards with Hibiclens or soapy water. If deep, treat as indicated
above under puncture wound with hot soaks and antibiotics.

Fishhook Removal

The first aid approach to an impaled fishhook is to tape it in place
and not try to remove it if there is any danger of causing damage to
nearby or underlying structures or if the patient is uncooperative. Cut
the fish line off the hook. Destroy triple hooks, but do not cut the hook

close to the skin with your wire cutters. This makes subsequent manipulation by the surgeon more difficult.

If you will be longer than 2 days from help, it is important to remove any impaled object, to include a fishhook, as such objects are a high risk for infection. And, since fishhooks are relatively easy to remove anyway, you may wish to do it yourself to prevent a long trip back to town and the doctor's waiting room.

There are three basic methods for removing a fishhook, which I refer to as "the good, the bad, and the ugly" techniques. I will let you decide which is which:

Push through, snip off method—While the technique seems straightforward, consider a few points: (1) Pushing the hook should not endanger underlying or adjacent structures. This limits the technique's usefulness, but it is still frequently an easy, quick method to employ. (2) Skin is not easy to push through. It is very elastic and will tent up over the barb as you try to push it through. Place side-cutting wire cutters, with jaws spread apart, over the point on the surface where you expect the hook point to punch through to hold the skin down while the barbed point punches its way to the surface. (3) This is a painful process and skin hurts when being poked from the bottom up, as much as from the top

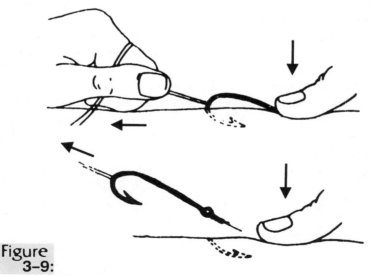

**Figure
 3-9:**

Press shank of hook against the
skin surface. B. Vigorously jerk hook along the skin surface.

down. Once committed, get the push through portion of this project over with in a hurry. (4) This adds a second puncture wound to the victim's anatomy. Cleanse the skin at the anticipated penetration site before shoving the hook through using soap or a surgical scrub. (5) When snipping the protruding point off, cover the wound area with your free hand to protect you and others from the flying hook point. Otherwise you may need to refer to the section on "removing foreign bodies from the eye" on page 36. The steps are simple: (1) Push the hook through. (2) Snip it off. (3) Back the barb-less hook out. (4) Treat the puncture wounds. If you do not have wire cutters, you may still use this technique, but be able to crush the barb flat enough that you will be able to back the hook out.

The string-jerk method—this is the most elegant of the methods. Fingers are loaded with fibrous tissue that tends to hinder a smooth hook removal. This technique works best in the back of the head, the shoulder, and most aspects of the torso, arms, and legs. It is highly useful and can be virtually painless, causing minimal trauma.

See Figure 3–9: (A) Loop a line, such as the fish line, around the hook, ensuring that this line is held flush against the skin. Pushing down on the eye portion of the hook helps disengage the hook barb, so that the quick pull (B) will jerk the hook free with minimal trauma. Many times a victim will ask "When are you going to pull it out?" after the job has been completed.

The dissection method—At times it just seems we are not to be so lucky and we have to resort to what will probably be a difficult experience for the victim and surgeon alike. This is the case of embedded triple hooks, a hook near the eye, or other situations when the above methods cannot be used. No person in his right mind would attempt this on his own if evacuation to a physician was at all possible. It is tedious, and without a local anesthetic such as injectable lidocaine, extremely painful.

The technique employs the use of either a sharp, thin blade or an 18-gauge or larger bore hypodermic needle. Examine a hook similar to the one that is embedded in the victim to note the bend in the shank and the location of the barb. You will need to slide the blade along the hook shank, cutting the strands of connective tissue so that the hook can be backed out. If using the needle, you will need to slide it along the hook and attempt to cover the barb with a hollow tube, thus shielding connective tissue strands from the barb, allowing the hook to be similarly backed out. This is an elegant method and can result in minimal tissue damage, with only the entry hole left. But it can take time and without local anesthesia the victim would have to be stoic. If available, inject a little 1% lidocaine from the Rx Injectable Medication Module. Practice using a piece of closed-cell foam sleeping pad, rather than human skin, prior to your trip in the bush.

Friction Blisters

Blisters can be prevented if immediate care is taken of any hot spot as soon as it develops. Generally a simple piece of tape placed directly over the hot spot will eliminate any friction causing the problem. An easily obtainable substance has revolutionized the prevention and care of friction blisters. The substance is Spenco 2nd Skin, available at most athletic supply and drug stores. Made from an inert, breathable gel consisting of 4% polyethylene oxide and 96% water, it has the feel and consistency of, well, most people would say snot. It comes in various sized sheets, sterile, and sealed in water-tight packages. It is very cool to the touch; in fact, large sheets are sold to cover infants to reduce a fever. It has three valuable properties that make it so useful: it will remove all friction between two moving surfaces (hence its use in prevention); it cleans and deodorizes wounds by absorbing blood, serum, or pus; and its cooling effect is very soothing, which aids in pain relief.

It comes between two sheets of cellophane. It must be held against the wound and for that purpose the same company produces an adhesive knit bandage. For prevention 2nd Skin can be applied with the cellophane attached and secured with the knit bandaging. For treatment of a hot spot, remove the cellophane from one side and apply this gooey side against the wound, again securing it with the knit bandaging. If a friction blister has developed, it will have to be lanced. Cleanse with soap or surgical scrub and open along an edge with a sharp blade. There is no advantage to making a small hole as opposed to a wide incision. Allow the skin covering to collapse by expressing the fluid, then apply a fully stripped piece of 2nd Skin. This is best done by removing the cellophane from one side, then apply it to the wound. Once it adheres to the skin surface, remove the cellophane from the outside edge. Over this you will need to place the adhesive knit. The bandage must be kept moist with clean water. The 2nd Skin should be replaced daily. If the skin cover is still covering the wound, it should be cut off after 2 days as the skin underneath is now less raw and the dead skin will start to decompose. Until you use it on a friction blister, you'll find it hard to believe how well 2nd Skin works!

The Spyroflex wound dressing in the Topical Bandaging Module is an excellent alternative to 2nd Skin. It can similarly absorb leaking fluid, provide direct protection to the raw skin, and eliminate friction. However, it does not provide the cooling effect of the 2nd Skin.

It makes good sense to coat all open blisters with triple antibiotic ointment. This acts as a barrier to prevent infection and the praxamne also helps to provide pain relief.

The old technique of blister care with rings of moleskin is seldom effective. Moleskin should be relegated to the Dark Ages of Wilderness Medicine.

Thermal Burns

As soon as possible remove the source of the burn. Quick immersion into cool water will help eliminate additional heat from scalding water or burning fuels and clothing. Do not over-cool the victim and cause hypothermia. If water is not available, suffocate the flames with clothing, sand, etc. Do not allow a victim to panic and run as this will fan the flames and increase the injury.

Treatment of burns depends upon the extent (percent of the body covered) and the severity (degree) of the injury. The percent of the body covered is estimated by referring to the "Rule of Nines," as indicated in Figure 3–10. An entire arm equals 9% of the body surface area, therefore the burn of just one side of the forearm would equal about 2%. The chest and back equal 18% and the abdomen and back equal 18%. The proportions are slightly different for small children, the head representing a larger percentage (18%) and the legs a smaller percentage (13.5%). Severity of burns is indicated by degree. First degree (superficial) will have redness and be dry and painful. Second degree (partial skin thickness) will be moist, painful, and have blister formation with reddened bases. Third degree (deep) involves the full thickness of the skin and extends into the subcutaneous tissue with char, loss of substance, or discoloration.

For purposes of field management, victims can be divided into three groups depending upon a combination of the extent and severity of the burn.

First degree burns, regardless of the extent, rarely require evacuation. The severe pain initially encountered in a first degree burn usually disappears within 24 hours. The patient's requirement for pain medication can range from ibuprofen 200 mg 4 tablets every 4 to 6 hours, Percogesic, 2 tablets every 3 to 4 hours, to Lorcet 10/650, 1 tablet every 3 to 4 hours. After a few doses, further pain medication is generally not re-

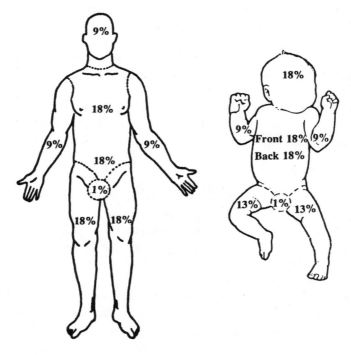

Figure 3-10: The "Rule of Nines" burn chart helps determine the percentage of a body covered by burns. Note the differences between an adult and an infant.

quired. Surface dressings are not indicated, but soothing relief of small burns can be obtained by either applying a Spenco 2nd Skin dressing or damp cloth.

Second degree burns covering less than 15% and third degree burns covering less than 10% of the body surface area do not require rapid evacuation, but should receive professional care. Provide pain medication as above. Cleanse the area with either a surgical scrub or non-medicated soap. Do not attempt to remove debris that is stuck to the burn site. Gently pat dry. The general consensus is to remove skin from blisters that have ruptured or that are blood filled. I find it best to initially leave the skin covering on the blister, removing it after 3 days. People generally feel better when you open turgid blisters with a long cut using a sharp blade. Apply Spenco 2nd Skin dressing and change twice daily. Second degree burns will slough the skin after 3 to 4 days. An unopened or covered blister surface will turn white in 3 days and frequently an ooze of pus may develop in the underlying blister fluid. If the underlying skin does not become red and swollen, this is a normal development. White moist dead skin should be cut away. If you have no ointment or dressings, leave a second or third degree burn alone. The surface of the blister, if it is drained, will dry out and slough off on its own. Either way, healing will take place in 2 weeks or less for a second degree burn. A third degree burn greater than half a square inch will require a skin graft to heal. Red swollen skin under and around the burn site probably indicates an infection. If this develops, provide antibiotics from the Rx Oral/Topical Medication Module such as Levaquin 500 mg once daily or from the Rx Injectable Module give Rocephin 500 mg intramuscular twice daily. Elevate the burned area to minimize the swelling.

A third degree burn greater than 10% and second degree burn greater than 15% of the total body surface area; any serious burn to the face; and any third degree burn of hands, feet, or genitals require urgent evacuation of the patient. Wound management is the least important part of the care of these patients. Burn wounds are sterile for the first 24 to 48 hours. Burn management is aimed at keeping the wound clean, reducing pain, and treating for shock.

An important aspect of treating for shock will be maintaining adequate fluid replacement. Generally patients with less than 20% of their body surface area burned can tolerate oral fluids very well. If they are not vomiting, those with between 20% and 30% of their body surface area involved can be resuscitated by drinking adequate fluids. This individual will be prone to go into shock. If the victim is vomiting, he will fall behind in fluid replacement.

The replacement fluid should initially consist of Gatorade diluted 1:1 with water or a mixture consisting of ½ teaspoon of salt and ½ teaspoon of baking soda in 1 quart of flavored, lightly sweetened water. Avoid the use of potassium-rich solutions (orange juice, apple juice) as serum potassium can raise to high levels during the first 24 hours. During the second day the oral fluids should be diluted Gatorade and lightly sweetened, flavored water (such as Wylers or dilute Tang). Push as much fluid during these 2 days as the patient can tolerate without becoming nauseous. Attempt to keep urine flow 50 to 100 ml (1⅔ ounce to 3⅓ ounce) per hour. Nausea can be suppressed with adequate pain management and the use of Atarax 25 to 50 mg every 6 hours from the Rx Oral/Topical Medication Module or Vistaril 25 to 50 mg by intramuscular injection every 4 hours as needed from the Rx Injectable Module. Pain relief will require Nubain 10 to 20 mg intramuscular or the nasally inhaled Stadol (see page 225) or the oral medications as tolerated. Patients who lapse into a coma during the first 48 hours will require intravenous fluids to save their lives. Physicians equipped with IV fluids are aware of the massive doses that are required to succeed at this point.

Starting the third day the patient should be given a moderately high carbohydrate diet, rich in protein. Approximately 200 mg of vitamin C and substantial vitamin B complex should be started daily. This would equal about 4 each One-A-Day multiple vitamin (Miles) or equivalent. Continue to push fluids.

Spenco 2nd Skin is the ideal burn dressing for these severe burns. It provides a breathable cover that is sterile and will exclude bacteria from the environment. It is also easily removed with whirlpool or gentle cleansing. Otherwise apply a topical dressing such as triple antibiotic ointment. Occlusive dressings must not be used. The ointment may be placed on thick gauze dressings that are then held against the wound with a single layer of gauze roll dressing. The wound should be cleaned daily, removing obviously dead tissue. This can be done with gentle scraping using a sterile gauze and clean water with a little Hibiclens surgical scrub added, about half an hour after proper pain medication has been provided. Lacking Hibiclens, use a very dilute soap solution. Elevate the burned area, if practical. Have the victim gently and regularly move the burned area as much as possible to minimize contraction of burn tissue across joints. This will only be a concern with long-term care lasting many weeks.

Avoid the use of oral or injectable antibiotics to prevent wound infection. If you suspect an infection has developed because the underlying tissue is becoming red and swollen, red streaks are traveling from the burn towards the heart, or the burn was grossly contaminated (such as from an explosion), use antibiotics as described above.

Human Bites

Unless group discipline has really degenerated, human bites are due to accidents such as falling and puncturing flesh with teeth. Bites within the victim's own mouth seldom become infected and are discussed in the section on lacerations (see page 58). Human bites to any other location of the body have the highest infection rate of any wound. Scrub vigorously with Hibiclens surgical scrub, soapy water, or any other antiseptic that you can find. Pick out broken teeth or other debris. Use the

Sawyer Extractor for 10 minutes, further use will not help. Coat the wound area with triple antibiotic ointment. Start the application of hot, wet compresses as described under puncture wounds. Start antibiotic with Rocephin 500 mg IM every 12 hours, or from the Rx Oral/Topical Module use Levaquin 500 mg once daily. Bite wounds to the hand are extremely serious and should be seen by a qualified hand surgeon as soon as possible.

Animal Bites

Animal bites tend to be either tearing or crushing injuries. Animal bite lacerations must be vigorously cleaned, but hot soaks need not be started initially. Some authorities state that bite lacerations should not be taped or sutured closed due to an increased incidence of wound infection. This has not been my personal experience, nor that of many ER physicians with whom I have discussed this problem. After vigorous wound cleansing I would close gaping wounds as described under *lacerations*. Puncture wounds should not be closed, only gaping wounds. Start antibiotic coverage immediately, as described in the section on human bites. The massive lacerations from a large animal bite, such as bear or puma injuries, are another matter. The entire goal of treatment is to stop the bleeding, treat for shock, and evacuate. You may need to close these massive lacerations to help control bleeding.

If an infection seems to start, treat as indicated in the section on wound infection on page 114 by removing the closures and starting hot soaks and antibiotics.

Treat crush injuries with cold packs and compressive dressings. Large lacerations can also be treated with compressive dressings. The ideal item would be a 6-inch elastic bandage. Cold sources can be chemical cold packs or the coldest water available, safely packaged in poly bottles or similar containers.

Refer to *rabies* (page 182).

Finger and Toe Problems

Ingrown Nail

This painful infection along the edge of a nail can, at times, be relieved with warm soaks. There are several maneuvers that can hasten healing however. One technique is a taping procedure, shown in Figure

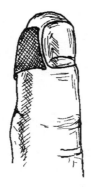
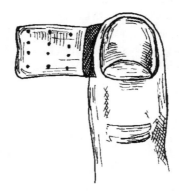

Figure 3–11: Apply tape to skin edge next to the nail and tug the skin away from the nail, fastening the tape down under the toe or finger.

3–11. A piece of strong tape (such as waterproof tape) is taped to the inflamed skin edge, next to—but not touching—the nail. The tape is fastened tightly to this skin edge with gentle, but firm pressure. By running the tape under the toe, the skin edge can be tugged away from the painful nail and thus relieve the pressure.

Another method is to shave the top of the nail by scraping it with a sharp blade until it is thin enough that it buckles upwards. This "breaks the arch" of the nail and allows the ingrown edge to be forced out of the inflamed groove along the side. The above techniques should be implemented at the first sign of irritation rather than once infection has developed, though even then they are effective. Provide antibiotic such as doxycycline 100 mg twice daily or Levaquin once daily.

Paronychia (Nail Base Infection)

An infection of the nail base (paronychia) is a very painful condition that should initially be treated with warm soaks, 15 minutes, every 2 hours, and the use of oral antibiotics such as doxycycline 100 mg twice daily or Levaquin 500 mg daily. Oral pain medication will also be necessary. If the lesion does not respond within 2 days, or if it seems to be getting dramatically worse, an aggressive incision with a sharp blade will

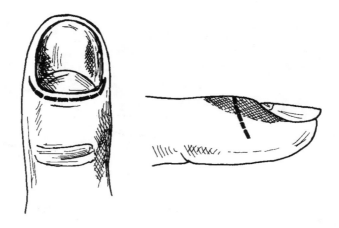

Figure 3-12: Paronychia, showing the incision required to drain the abscess.

be necessary, as shown in Figure 3–12. This wound will bleed freely. Allow it to do so. Change bandages as necessary, and continue the soaks and medications as described under *abscess*.

Felon

A deep infection of a fingertip is called a felon. It results in a tense, tender finger pad. Soaking a felon prior to surgery, unlike other infections, does not help and only increases the pain. Treatment is effected by a very aggressive incision, called a fish–mouth incision, made along the tip of the finger from one side to the other and extending deep to the bone. (See Figure 3–13).

An alternate incision is a through–and–through stab wound going under the finger bone, from one side to the other. A gauze or sterile plastic strip is then inserted through the wound to promote drainage of the pus from the felon.

The pain is severe and not helped by local injection of lidocaine. But relief is quick in coming as pressure from the pus build-up is then alleviated. Allow this wound to bleed freely. Soak in warm water for 15 minutes, every 2 hours until drainage ceases (about 3 days). Give pain medication about one hour prior to your surgical procedure, using the strongest that you have in your kit. Simultaneously start the victim on

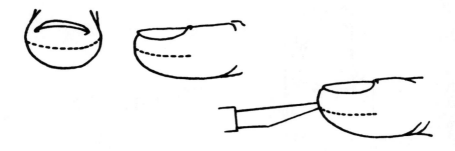

Figure 3-13: Felon, showing the incision required to drain the abscess.

antibiotic such as Levaquin 500 once daily, doxycycline 100 mg twice daily, or Rocephin 500 mg IM twice daily.

Blood Under the Nail

Blood under a fingernail or toenail, called subungual hematoma is generally caused by a blow to the digit involved. The accumulation of blood under a nail can be very painful. Relieve this pressure by twirling the sharp point of a blade through the nail (using the lightest pressure possible) until a hole is produced and draining effected. This is a painless procedure and the tip of the blade should not enter the nailbed, only the pocket of blood under the nail. Soak in cool water to promote continual drainage of this blood. The finger may hurt from the contusion still, however, so additional pain treatment with Percogesic 1 or 2 tablets every 4 hours or Lorcet 10/650 1 tablet every 4 to 6 hours, may also be useful. Antibiotic use is not necessary.

Wound Infection and Inflammation

Lacerations that have been cleaned and either sutured, taped, or stapled together will generally become slightly inflamed. Inflammation is part of the healing process and does not indicate infection, yet the appearance is similar. It is a matter of degree. Inflammation has slight swelling and red color. The hallmarks of infection are: swelling, warmth to touch, reddish color, and pain. Pus oozing out of a wound is another clue. If the cut has a red swelling that extends beyond ¼ inch from the wound edge, infection has probably started.

The method of treatment of wound infection is quite simple. Remove some of the tapes (sutures or staples) and allow the wound to open and drain. Apply warm, moist compresses for 15 to 20 minutes every 2 hours. This will promote drainage of the wound and increase the local circulation, thus bringing large numbers of friendly white blood cells and fibroblasts into the area. The fibroblast tries to wall off the infection and prevent the further spread of germs. Once an infection has obviously started, the use of an antibiotic will be helpful, but not always essential. From the Rx Oral/Topical Module use the Levaquin 500 mg once daily. If the Rx Injectable Module is available, use the Rocephin 500 mg twice daily IM or 1,000 mg once daily IM.

Abscess

An abscess (boil, furuncle) is a pocket of pus (white blood cells), germs, and red blood cells that have been contained by an envelope of scar tissue produced by fibroblasts. This protects the body from the further spread of germs. It is part of the body's strong natural defense against invasion by bacteria. Conversely, many antibiotics cannot penetrate into the abscess cavity very well. The cure of an abscess is surgical. It must be opened and drained. There are two basic ways in which this can happen. First, moist warm soaks will not only aid in abscess formation, but will also aid in bringing the infection to the surface and cause the infection to "ripen," even open and drain on its own. An abscess can be very painful and this opening period very prolonged. Once the abscess is on the surface it is generally better to open it using a technique called "incision and drainage" or I&D. The ideal instrument for an I&D is a thin, sharp blade. Use the blade to penetrate the surface skin and open the cavity with minimal pressure on the wound. Abscesses are very painful, primarily because of the pressure within them. A person coming into a doctor's office with a painful abscess would expect to have it anesthetized before opening. Injections into these areas only add to the pain. The best anesthesia is to cool the wound area. In the field an ice cube or application of an instant cold pack will help provide some anesthesia. A person with a painful abscess will usually let you try the knife as they can become desperate for pain relief. The relief that they get when the pressure is removed is immediate, even without cooling. Coat the skin surface around the abscess with triple antibiotic ointment from the non-Rx Topical Bandaging Module to protect the skin from the bacteria that are draining from the wound. Spread of infection from these bacteria is unlikely, however, unless the skin is abraded or otherwise broken.

Cellulitis

Cellulitis is a very dangerous and rapidly progressive skin infection that results in red, painful swelling of the skin without pus or blister formation. The lesion spreads by the hour, with streaks of red progressing ahead of the swelling toward the heart. This represents the travel of infection along the lymphatic system and is frequently called "blood poisoning" in the vernacular. While lymphatic spread is not strictly blood poisoning, cellulitis does frequently lead to generalized blood poisoning (septicemia) and can cause the development of chills, fever, and other symptoms of generalized profound infection, such as lethargy and even shock. Very dangerous and virulent germs are responsible. Strong antibiotics are necessary. The application of local heat is very helpful. Old time remedies included the use of various "drawing salves," but nothing works better than local hot compresses. Local heat increases the circulation of blood into the infected area, bringing white cells that will kill the bacteria directly and also produce antibodies to aid in killing the germs. The infection fighters, and the walling-off process of the fibroblasts, will hopefully contain and destroy the infection. When this walling off process succeeds, an abscess is formed (see next section). If the Rx Injectable Module is available, give Rocephin 500 mg IM twice daily. Or, if only the Rx Oral/Topical Module is available, give the doxycycline 100 mg twice daily or Levaquin 500 mg once daily.

Skin Rash

A rash is a frequent outdoor problem. At times a rash is associated with certain diseases and can help in the diagnosis. If the patient is feverish, or obviously ill, review the sections on Lyme disease, Rocky Mountain spotted fever, typhoid fever, syphilis, meningococcal meningitis, strep throat, measles, and mononucleosis. Many infections that cause rash are viral and will not respond to antibiotic. But in the wilderness, with no professional medical help available, rash associated with symptoms of illness, particularly fever and aching, should be empirically treated with antibiotic such as the doxycycline 100 mg twice daily for at least 2 days beyond the defervescence (loss of fever). Some of the above infections require longer antibiotic treatment, so it should be continued as indicated if there is a probability that you are dealing with one of them.

Localized rashes without fever are usually due to superficial skin infections, fungal infections, or allergic reactions. Itch can be treated with antihistamine or any pain medication. The Non-Rx Oral Medication Module has diphenhydramine 25 mg as an antihistamine. One capsule (2 in severe cases) every 6 hours will help with itch from nearly any cause. As itch travels over the same nerves that carry the sensation of pain, any pain medication can also help with itch. Warm soaks generally make itch and rash worse and should be avoided, unless there is evidence of deep infection (see *cellulitis* and *abscess* above). It is hard to do better than diphenhydramine with regard to oral antihistamine effect, but it should be noted that Atarax (in the Rx Oral/Topical Module) and the same medication in injectable form, Vistaril (in the Rx Injectable Module), also have antihistamine action and can be used for itch. Also soothing to either a non-weeping lesion or a blistered and weeping lesion is the application of a piece of Spenco 2nd Skin from the Topical Bandaging Module. Cool compresses will also sooth a rash.

If it is a moist, weeping lesion, wet soaks of dilute epsom salts, boric acid, or even table salt will help dry the lesion (this includes poison ivy, poison oak, and poison sumac). If it is a dry scaly rash, an ointment works the best, much better than a gel, lotion, or cream. Blistered rashes are treated best with creams, lotions, or gels. Specific types of rash require specific types of topical medications, however.

Fungal Infection

A fungal rash is commonly encountered in the groin, in the armpit, in skin folds, on the scrotum, under a woman's breasts, and around the rectum. Rashes can range from bright red to almost colorless, but are generally at least dull red and frequently have small satellite spots near the major portion of confluent rash. Fungal infections are very slow in spreading, with the lesions becoming larger over a period of weeks to months. Body ring worm is a circular rash with a less intense center area (*caution:* see *Lyme disease,* page 180). Fungal rashes should be treated with a specific antifungal, such as the clotrimazole 2% cream from the Non-Rx Topical Bandaging Module. Apply a thin coat twice daily. Good results should be obtained within 2 weeks for "jock itch," but athlete's foot and body ring worm may take 4 weeks. If so, continue treatment until all evidence of rash is gone, then continue treatment once daily for an additional 3 weeks. If no improvement has been made, the diagnosis may have been wrong or the fungus is refractory to your medication. From the Rx Oral Medication Module Diflucan 150 mg daily will destroy most body surface fungal infections, but it is included in only a small quantity for primary use in the treatment of vaginitis.

Allergic Dermatitis

The hallmarks of an *allergic dermatitis* are vesicles, or small blisters, on red, swollen, and very itchy skin. A line of these blisters clinches the diagnosis of allergic, or contact dermatitis. The most common reasons are poison ivy, poison sumac, and poison oak. Contact with caterpillars, millipedes, and many plants—even such innocent species as various evergreens—can induce allergic or toxic skin reactions. A toxic reaction to a noxious substance, such as from certain insects and plants, is treated like an allergic dermatitis. First aid treatment is a thorough cleansing with soap and water. Further treatment is with diphenhydramine 25 mg every 6 hours from the Non-Rx Oral Medication Module and twice daily applications of hydrocortisone cream 1% from the Topical Bandaging Unit. Weeping lesions can be treated with wet soaks as mentioned above. An occlusive plastic dressing will allow the rather weak 1% hydrocortisone to work much better.

The Rx Oral/Topical Medication Module has two very effective medications to treat this problem. Continue use of the diphenhydramine, but add Decadron 4 mg tablets, 1 daily for 5 to 7 days and apply the Topicort 0.25% ointment in place of the hydrocortisone cream. A thin coat twice daily without an occlusive plastic dressing should work rapidly.

Stinging nettle causes a severe irritation that can be instantly eliminated by the application of "GI jungle juice," a mixture of 75% DEET insect repellent and 25% isopropyl (rubbing) alcohol. I discovered this neat trick the hard way (accidentally) while camping in fields of the stuff along the Cape Fear River in North Carolina. Since mentioning this in the first edition of *Wilderness Medicine* in 1979, many others in contact with this plant have confirmed the treatment's instantaneous effectiveness.

Bacterial Skin Rash

A common bacterial superficial skin infection causing a rash is *impetigo*. The normal appearance of this condition is reddish areas around pus-filled blisters, which are frequently crusty and scabbed. The lesions spread rapidly over a period of days. The skin is generally not swollen underneath the lesions. It often starts around the nose and on the buttocks, spreads rapidly from scratching, and can soon appear anywhere on the body. Early lesions appear as small pimples, which form crusts within 12 to 24 hours. Lesions should be cleaned with surgical soap (or hydrogen peroxide) and then covered with an application of triple antibiotic ointment. Avoid placing bandages on these lesions as the germs can spread under the tape.

Bacterial skin infections generally must be treated with prescription antibiotics. From the Rx Oral/Topical Medication Module give Levaquin once daily. The Rx Injectable Medication Module contains Rocephin, which would be ideal for this condition. Give 500 mg IM once daily. Treatment of cellulitis and abscess, forms of deep skin infections, are discussed on pages 116 and 115.

See page 56 for treatment of *cold sores* and *lip or mouth lesions.*

Seabather's Eruption

"Seabather's eruption" is the term used for the sudden onset of a very itchy rash associated with swimming. In south Florida and the Caribbean it is caused by larvae of the thimble jellyfish (*Linuche unguiculata*) or by the larvae of the sea anemone, *Edwardsella lineata*. The latter was shown to be responsible for thousands of cases on Long Island, New York. Welts (urticaria) or a fine red rash or pimply rash appear within 24 hours of exposure to ocean water, normally in areas covered by bathing suits. The tiny larvae are trapped next to the skin within the bathing suit and discharge nematocysts that cause the disease. Additional symptoms frequently associated with this rash include fever, chills, weakness, and headache, as the larvae penetrate the skin and cause illness. In south Florida the occurrence is from March to August, with a peak of outbreaks in May. In Long Island waters the outbreaks occur from mid-August until the end of the swimming season in early September. These outbreaks are episodic with very few cases some years and thousands of cases during peak years.

Treatment consists of topical corticosteroid (1% hydrocortisone cream from the Non-RX Topical Bandaging Module applied four times daily or 0.25% Topicort ointment from the Rx Oral/Topical Module applied twice daily) and antihistamine (diphenhydramine 25 mg from the Non-Rx Oral Medication Module four times a day). Swimmers should remove their bathing suits and shower as soon as possible after leaving the water. And swimming at a nude beach doesn't protect you from this just because you are not wearing a bathing suit.

Orthopedic Injuries

Concepts of Orthopedic Care

The above table will refer you to general management principles and to diagnosis and treatment plans by anatomical region.

Orthopedics includes the study of bone, joint, and muscle function and disorders. This section establishes basic protocols for the assessment and care of orthopedic disorders. General concepts of care will be followed by a systematic assessment by anatomical region with suggested care plans.

Concepts of Orthopedic Care

Muscle Pain—No Acute Injury

Muscle aches can arise from chronic inflammation disorders such as lupus and fibromyalgia, but the discussion here will be limited to those conditions that might reasonably arise on a wilderness trek.

When associated with a fever, consider an infectious basis for the pain. Without a reasonable method of diagnosis, it would be best to treat with both an antibiotic and appropriate pain medication. Even in North America, several serious conditions can present in this manner that require urgent treatment, such as Rocky Mountain Spotted Fever. Regardless of cause, it is appropriate to start ibuprofen 200 mg tablets, 2 to 4 tablets each dose, repeated every 6 hours, for fever and muscle ache.

While it's best to have a physician see the patient and to draw the appropriate lab tests before commencing antibiotics, if you are more than 2 days journey from treatment, start the doxycycline 100 mg twice daily. If you might be treating Lyme disease, this treatment will need to be continued for at least 2 weeks (see page 180).

Under conditions of heat stress, heavy exertion causing sweating, diarrhea, vomiting, or the use of diuretics causing increased urine output, a cause for muscle cramping is electrolyte abnormality. Appropriate fluid and electrolyte replacement is necessary as discussed on page 82.

Overuse syndromes cause pain in muscles that go beyond the mild ache you are accustomed to feeling after a workout at the gym. While it is possible to suddenly tear muscles with sudden movements, significant pain that starts gradually or after the exercise is over, can represent pain caused by a tendinitis, spasm caused by a pinched nerve, or significant inflammation in the muscle. The treatment for these conditions is the same as that employed for tendinitis as described in that section. Additionally, the use of a muscle relaxer is of benefit. From the Non-Rx Oral Medication Module take Percogesic 2 tablets every 6 hours or from the Rx Oral/Topical Module use Atarax 25 mg every 6 hours. These medications can be used in addition to the others prescribed for tendinitis unless the condition is relatively mild when the use of Percogesic alone should suffice.

Muscle Pain—Acute Injury

Pain occurs immediately after a significant muscle injury, a contusion or strain being the general cause. RICE is the acronym that applies here: Rest, Ice, Compress, Elevate. An elastic bandage, cold stream water, elevation of a limb, and rest may not all be possible, but they comprise the initial treatment. The application of cold is the most important, though be careful not to cause freezing injury.

Contusions cause bleeding into the surrounding muscle tissue through the rupture of small blood vessels. RICE will minimize the bleeding and local swelling. Strains on muscles result in either microscopic muscle fiber tears or muscle mass tears. These are graded as Grade I (microscopic) to Grade IV (total tear of a muscle). Grades II and III are partial tears of a muscle mass. A total tear would require surgical repair. All will be treated alike in the wilderness setting. Initially use RICE, as indicated above. If significant swelling of the muscle occurs, consider that you are dealing with a Grade III or IV tear, and continue RICE for 2 days. Otherwise use RICE for the first 24 hours.

The next step in treating significant muscle injury would be the application of local heat. In the case of minor injuries, apply the next day. For more serious injuries, delay the use of heat for 2 days. Continue the use of the compression dressing. Splint or sling as necessary for comfort. Decrease activity to a level where the pain is tolerable.

A full rupture of a muscle body will generally result in a bulging of the muscle mass and a loss of strength during the late recovery period. This may not be noticeable at first as the swelling would initially be attributed to local bleeding and the pain would restrict use. Once the pain is gone, continued swelling, especially after several weeks have passed, is probably due to a significant muscle tear or a ruptured tendon. This should be repaired when possible, but it is not a reason for an urgent evacuation.

Joint Pain—No Acute Injury

Pain in the joint without history of injury is generally due to arthritis, bursitis, or tendinitis. Without a history of previous arthritis the latter two are the more likely diagnosis, but the treatment is the same for all three. The most common reason for tendon or joint inflammation is over-use. French trappers frequently complained of Achilles tendinitis while snowshoeing, which they aptly termed "mal de racquette." Persons hammering, chopping wood, or playing tennis are familiar with "tennis elbow" (epicondylitis of the elbow). Tendinitis can occur in the thumb, wrist—in fact any tendon in the body can become inflamed with overuse. Joints similarly become inflamed with repetitious activity or even unusual compression. Cave explorers and canoeists will, on occasion, encounter a patellar bursitis of the knees, and many people have formed bursitis flare-ups in a shoulder after repetitive arm actions. Rafters, kayakers, and canoeists can develop tendinitis in the forearm due to the over-use of flexor tendons of the wrist.

Treatment of these conditions must include altering the activity that seems to have caused it. By changing a grip on an oar, using paddles with a different pitch to the blades, altering a movement to avoid generating additional pain, the victim can try to alleviate the discomfort and avoid inflaming it more. Prior to an activity the application of heat to the sore area helps. Immediately after aggravating the condition, applying cold is a benefit. Within an hour return to a local heat application and continue this during the evenings. Applying a cream such as Aspercream (other brand names are Myoflex and Mobisyl) with a dry heat might help a tendinitis as the active ingredient trolamine salicylate (10% concentration) penetrates the skin and provides local anti-inflammatory action. Sports creams that feel warm, such as Icy-Hot, simply irritate the skin surface to cause an increased blood flow and thus provide warmth to the area. They do not have an anti-inflammatory effect and they do not provide any benefit over the application of heat. This does not mean that these creams do not have a potentially valuable role here. It is very difficult to apply hot soaks in a wilderness setting and these creams can serve the purpose.

If hot compresses seem to aggravate the pain, switch to a cold compress technique. Avoid making any movements which seem to cause the most pain for 5 to 7 days. Splinting may help during this period. Avoid non-use of the shoulder for longer than 2 weeks as it is prone to adhesion formation and loss of function can result.

The best medication for chronic joint pain is the ibuprofen from the Non-Rx Oral Medication Module due to its anti-inflammatory action. Four tablets every 6 hours will aid in joint and tendon pain. From the Rx Oral/Topical Medication Module one could use the Decadron 4 mg, given once daily for 7 days for joint inflammation. The Lorcet 10/650 may be necessary for pain relief, but it has no anti-inflammation activity like the ibuprofen.

Joint Pain—Acute Injury

Immediately after a joint injury, we all want to evaluate the injury, determine how serious it is, and figure out how or if the injury may change our expedition plans. Frankly, making a precise diagnosis usually isn't possible initially, so our approach to the acute joint injury must be to look at methods of treatment and potential long-term care. The discussion on orthopedic injuries in this book considers the body by region, not by precise diagnosis of injury. Nevertheless, we must try to have some understanding of what might have happened, make an accurate prognosis early in the event, and minimize the damage while keeping the victim as functional as possible.

Unusual stress across a joint can result in damage to supporting ligaments. Ordinarily this is a temporary stretching damage, but in severe cases rupture of ligaments or even fracture of bones or tears of cartilage can result. These injuries are serious problems and may require surgical repair. This is best done immediately, but can be safely delayed 2 to 3 months. Fractures entering the joint space may result in long-term joint pain and subsequent arthritis. Cartilage tears do not heal themselves, unlike ligament, tendon, and bone damage. These frequently cause so much future pain and instability that surgical correction is required.

Proper care of joint injuries must be started immediately. RICE—rest, ice, compression, and elevation—again forms the basis of good first aid management. Cold should be applied for the first 2 days, as continuously as possible. Then apply heat for 20 minutes or longer, 4 times daily. Cold decreases the circulation, which lessens bleeding and swelling. Heat increases the circulation, which then aids the healing process. This technique applies to all injuries including muscle contusions and bruises.

Elevate the involved joint, if possible. Wrap with elastic bandage or cloth tape to immobilize the joint and provide moderate support once ambulation or use of the joint begins. Take care that the wrappings are not so tightly applied that they cut off the circulation.

Use crutches or other support to take enough weight off an injured ankle and knee to the point that increased pain is not experienced. The patient should not use an injured joint if use causes pain, as this indicates further strain on the already stressed ligaments or fracture. Conversely, if use of the injured part does not cause pain, additional damage is not being done even if there is considerable swelling. If the victim must walk on an injured ankle or knee, and doing so causes considerable pain, then support it the best way possible (wrapping, crutches, decreased carrying load, tight boot for ankle injury) and realize that further damage is being done, but that in your opinion the situation warrants such a sacrifice.

While compression is good for an acute injury, too much could cut off circulation and must be avoided. If an ankle is injured, the boot can provide needed compression, but remove it if the pain becomes intolerable. A boot can always be put back on a swollen ankle by undoing the laces and just wrapping them around the boot circumference rather than using the eyelets.

Pain medications may be given as needed, but elevation and decreased use will provide considerable pain relief. See also fractures below.

Fractures

A fracture is a medical term meaning a broken bone. It is not true that "if you can move the part it is not broken." Pain will prevent some movement, but this does not aid in the diagnosis between a fracture and a contusion. Fractures may consist of a single crack in the bone and be rather stable or have many cracks and pieces and consequently be very unstable. There may be no way of telling which is present, or even if a fracture is there at all, without an x-ray. Deformity indicates either a fracture or contusion with soft tissue bleeding if located in the middle of a long bone area, or a possible dislocation or severe sprain with or without a fracture if located at a joint. The hallmark of a fracture is point tenderness or pain to touch over the site of the break. Swelling over the break site is further evidence of a fracture. Another way to deduce the presence of a fracture is to apply gentle torsion or compression to the bone in question with either technique causing increased pain at the fracture site.

Each fracture has several critical aspects in its management to consider: (1) correct loss of circulation or nerve damage due to deformity of the fracture; (2) prevent the induction of infection if the skin is broken at or near the fracture site; (3) prevent further soft tissue damage; and (4) obtain reasonable alignment of bone fragments so that adequate healing takes place. The nonskilled practitioner is limited to the first three management techniques.

The first aid approach to a fracture is to "splint them as they lie." This is not an appropriate response in remote areas. Straighten gross deformities of angulated fractures with gentle in-line traction, as in Figure 4–1. Before straightening, check the pulses beyond the fracture site on both sides of the victim and check for any abnormality of sensation. After correcting the angulation the circulation should improve. As arteries and veins are hollow tubes, their lumen will stretch and narrow if they are forced to bend around a corner, thus decreasing blood flow. When this bend is eliminated, the vessel will return to its normal size and blood flow will improve. As the person could be in shock, it might be difficult to feel the pulses on either side. A comparison is much more accurate than attempting to evaluate the circulation by examination of the injured side only.

Grossly angulated fractures also cause sharps ends of bone to project against the skin surface. Even with careful padding, jostling along during an evacuation may cause one of these bone spicules to penetrate the skin surface, causing an open fracture, increasing the chance of serious wound and bone infection.

The chance of causing harm while straightening an angulated fracture would be extremely low. It is possible for a blood vessel or nerve to become trapped within the fracture site, but gentle repositioning into slight deformity should correct this.

Pad splints well to prevent skin damage. Pneumatic splints are avail-

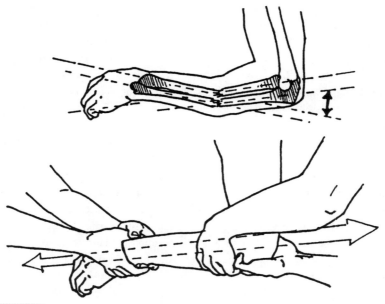

Figure 4-1: Use traction-in-line to straighten grossly angulated fractures. This technique is not meant to perfectly align the bone ends; it is only meant to eliminate gross deformity.

able from many outfitters. Fracture splinting is generally well covered in first aid courses. Such a course should be taken before any major expedition into the bush. Improvisation is the name of the game in fracture immobilization and having an adequate first aid course provides one with information upon which to improvise. In general, splint fractures to immobilize the joint above and below the fracture site.

Any wound in the skin near a broken bone increases the chance of a bone infection. Follow the principles of thorough wound cleansing as indicated on page 91.

With proper splinting the pain involved with a fracture will decrease dramatically. Provide pain medication when possible. Pain control is discussed on page 30. The non-Rx Percogesic or Rx Atarax can be given to aid in muscle spasm control.

At times there will be uncertainty about whether a fracture exists. When in doubt, splint and treat for pain, avoiding the use of the involved part. Within a few days the pain will have diminished and the crisis may be over. If not, the suspicion of a fracture will loom even larger.

Open Fracture

Even a laceration or puncture wound near a broken bone is a cause for alarm. Such a wound can allow bacteria into the fracture site, causing a serious bone infection. This wound requires aggressive cleansing as indicated on page 91. The wound should not be closed as this increases the chance of infection. Wet dressings are best over an open wound. Soak the sterile dressing in sterile water, cover with a clean dry dressing. Change this dressing twice daily.

If a piece of bone is protruding from the skin, the break is called an "open fracture." The first aid approach is to splint in position and cover with a sterile dressing. In a remote area this approach will not work. This wound will require aggressive irrigation with surgical scrub or soap as described on page 91–92.

The aggressiveness of this cleansing action should be done in such a manner as not to cause further damage, but the area must be free of foreign particulate matter and as antiseptic as possible. Cover the wound with triple antibiotic ointment. Protect with sterile gauze dressings, with enough pressure to control bleeding only. Straighten the gross angulation of the fracture with gentle in-line traction. This will cause the protruding bone to disappear under the skin surface, unless the fragment is loose from the main bone. Allow this wound to remain open and dress as indicated above.

In all cases of a laceration or puncture wound near a fracture, place the victim on oral antibiotics when available. From the Rx Oral/Topical Medication Module use the Levaquin 500 mg daily. However, if the Rx Injectable unit is carried, give the Rocephin 500 mg IM twice daily. Continue the medication until the patient is evacuated or the medication runs out.

Diagnosis and Care Protocols

The diagnosis of these injuries will be difficult due to lack of experience or benefit of x-ray equipment. Uncertainties of diagnosis will exist and therefore a systematic approach to the evaluation and treatment of the injured patient has to be developed that will handle most common injuries appropriately.

The orthopedic evaluation is made easier because human beings have equal sides that can be compared. Take the clothing off both the injured and normal sides and compare, weather permitting. Look for swelling or different configuration. When examining the injured side, touch lightly. A fracture or sprain is very tender and will not require hard poking to elicit obvious pain. Swelling is from local bleeding, which a fracture will almost always cause. Several days after the injury a bruise may appear near it, or lower on the person. Gravity as well as various muscle groups and local anatomy can cause this spilled blood to migrate to a place on the surface different from the injury site. This does not mean that the injury is spreading; it just represents the displacement of blood and part of the reabsorption process of healing. Don't be concerned about the appearance of bruising and its spread in the days after the injury.

Head

Lacerations of the scalp or face result in massive bleeding, the care of which is discussed on page 99. Internal head injuries range from insignificant to lethal. Check the level of consciousness as per page 13. Urgent evacuation is necessary for anyone who has any of the following:

- Unconsciousness for more than 2 minutes
- Debilitating headache
- Loss of coordination or garbled speech
- Persistent nausea and vomiting
- Bruising behind the ears (a sign of skull fracture)

- Bruising around the eyes (a sign of skull fracture)
- Decrease in vision
- Clear fluid draining from nose and/or ears (possible spinal fluid)
- Seizures
- Relapse into unconsciousness.

Suspect a neck injury in anyone with a head injury. On most trips it is prudent to seek medical care for anyone who has been knocked unconscious for even a brief moment. They can walk and assist in their own evacuation if there is no apparent spine injury. If the patient is not thinking clearly, or has any of the above signs, immobilize the neck and entire spine. Initially this may have to be done on the ground, with them lying down and using hand traction to stabilize their head and neck.

A head-injured patient will frequently vomit. To avoid aspirating this into his lungs, place him face down, with face turned to one side, or sit the patient up with his head elevated to 30°. This position may also decrease some of the headache associated with head injury.

While the patient is kept awake for neurological assessments of levels of consciousness in civilization, if the evacuation will take a long time (several days), allow the person to fall asleep. While asleep the brain has its best chance to control its own swelling.

While the use of pain and antinausea medication might alter the mental status and are avoided in urban first aid care, in a remote area during long-term care, it makes sense to use these medications. It is best to use the mildest medication necessary for relief. Refer to *pain management* (page 30) and *nausea management* (page 68).

If you detect improvement in the symptoms over the next 2 days, the prognosis is very good.

Neck

Examination of the neck is a critical task to help preserve the spinal cord from injury if the neck is unstable. Without moving the neck, gently palpate along the spinous process to elicit point tenderness in the conscious patient. No point tenderness will generally mean no significant bone damage to the neck. In an unconscious patient with head trauma, treat as if the neck is fractured. Splint carefully for maximal immobilization. If the neck is at an odd angle, it should be straightened with gentle traction-in-line, by pulling steadily and slowly on the head along the line in which you find the neck. Move the neck to a neutral position with the spine in a line. This is a maneuver taught by wilderness first aid classes. Practice before attempting.

Patients should not be allowed to move, nor should they be lifted or transported without careful immobilization of the neck. The best technique for initial cervical immobilization is gentle but firm control by a person holding the patient's head. Remind the victim to remain still. Eventually this firm control can be replaced with a cervical collar or rolled ensolite pad or other soft material. The Sam Splint can be molded into a cervical collar, as shown in Figure 4–2. To adequately prevent neck injury, the cervical collar will have to be augmented with total body immobilization.

If no point tenderness is claimed by the conscious victim, but generalized pain and spasm of the neck muscles are present, the victim may be suffering a severe sprain. A neck brace made of a towel or other rolled cloth can help with the long-term treatment. Local warmth will help relax these muscles. Pain medication and muscle relaxants are useful in curing a neck sprain and spasm. It can take weeks for this injury to cease hurting.

Spine

The neurological assessment of potential neck injury includes assessment of the entire spine. For a neurological check ask the patient if

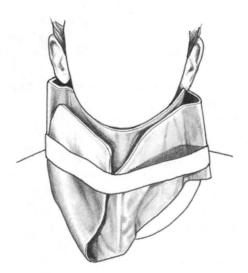

Figure 4–2: Sam Splint molded into a cervical collar. The vertical creases make the splint rigid.

there is any numbness or tingling anywhere on the body. Check grip strength on both sides and the ability to wiggle toes and flex feet up and down. Check the entire spine by palpating along the spinous processes looking for any point tenderness. If the above examination is questionable, or even if the trauma seems severe, both neck and spinal immobilization are in order. Having a rescuer maintain firm hand control of the victim's neck will be necessary until the patient has been placed upon a suitable rigid stretcher. Rigid stretchers are very difficult to improvise and moving people upon them even more difficult. While *Medicine for the Backcountry* (The Globe Pequot Press) goes into great detail in describing this technique, these skills require practice.

Ensure that the patient has been securely tied into the litter before you tie down the head. If the body shifts while the head is tied down, any damage present in the neck could increase.

In an urban environment, this is the end of the neck/spine story. The patient remains fastened rigidly to a stretcher until the emergency department physician has taken tests and made the determination that she can be removed. This may take several agonizing hours. I said agonizing, because even a normal person will hurt like crazy when attached to a rigid stretcher or back board. It's almost a self-fulfilling prophecy. If the patient didn't have back trouble when she was fastened down, she will when she is released. A recent study had 21 healthy volunteers (who had never experienced any back problems) placed in standard backboard immobilization for 30 minutes and found that 100% had pain during that period, with 55% grading it moderate to severe, and 29% developed additional symptoms after release during the following 48 hours.*

Especially in a remote area setting, it will be important to reassess the spine to ensure that continued immobilization is really necessary. This is difficult if even normal people will develop back pain after a short time on the board. You will have to use common sense. Inability to move an extremity or loss of sensation, without an orthopedic injury in that limb, must cause a high suspicion of spinal cord injury. But if these signs and symptoms are not present and you become convinced that you are dealing with only a sore muscle problem in the back, not a broken or disrupted spine, then the spine may be cleared—a term meaning let them out of the rigid support. Continued partial support with a soft

---

* Chan D., Goldber R., Tasone A., Harmon S., and Chan L. *The effect of spinal immobilization on healthy volunteers.* Ann EmergMed. January 1994; 23:48–51.

foam pad around the neck or even a back brace made of ensolite foam wrapped around the patient might make sense. Then again, it might not. It's a judgement call based upon the severity of the injury and resulting symptoms.

Collarbone

Evaluate for pain to palpation along the collarbone (clavicle). Separations of the clavicle from the sternum (breastbone), fractures of the clavicle, and separations of the shoulder can all be treated similarly with a sling and swathe, shown in Figure 4–3.

The clavicle frequently fractures in the mid-portion. Proper reduction will occur if the shoulders are held back, like those of a Marine at attention. A figure eight (Figure 4–4) will maintain this position. A stoop shoulder position will allow too much override of the fracture parts.

A fracture of the clavicle at the end near the shoulder may be hard to hold in proper position. In children there is a sleeve of tissue at this location that aids in holding the proper alignment. In adults this tissue is missing and even surgical pinning may be required for optimal healing.

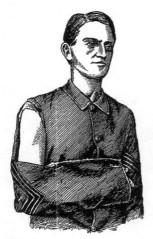 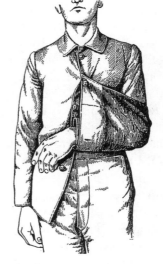

Figure 4–3:

A sling and swath will protect the injured shoulder and decrease pain in the recently fractured clavicle. This system can be duplicated by pinning the forearm to the front of a shirt. Use a sling without swath if there is a danger of the person slipping off a hill or falling into water.

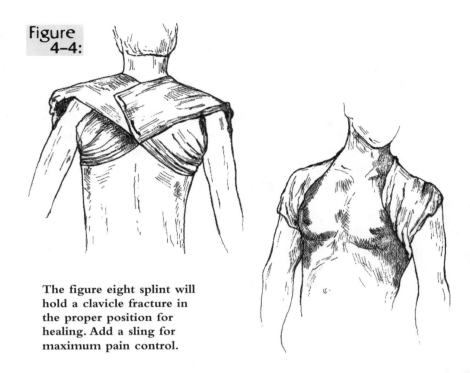

Figure 4-4:

The figure eight splint will hold a clavicle fracture in the proper position for healing. Add a sling for maximum pain control.

However, even in the adult this fracture may be treated adequately, usually with a sling.

A fracture of the clavicle at the end near the breastbone (sternum) is best reduced and held in position with a figure eight splint. In any clavicle fracture the use of a sling will aid greatly in decreasing pain. The sling can be eliminated in two weeks, but the figure eight splint should be kept on for 3 to 4 weeks, or until there is no pain over the fracture site with free movement of the shoulder.

Shoulder

Shoulder separations are classified as Grade I to Grade III, depending upon the severity. Grade I has tenderness over the acromio-clavicular joint (see Figure 4–5), representing a strain of the ligaments but with no disruption or tear. A Grade II is a rupture of the two acromio-clavicular ligaments, while a Grade III is disruption of both acromio-clavicular ligaments as well as the coraco-clavicular ligament. The latter case will allow elevation of the clavicle as the entire suspension of the shoulder has been disrupted. There is no strong evidence that Grade III separations do better with surgery than without if the patient is willing to accept slight deformity at the end of the clavicle. Functionally the patient should do fine by treating with an arm sling for 3 to 6 weeks for comfort with mobilization of the shoulder as early as possible and return to activity.

Shoulder dislocations are separations of the humerus (the long bone of the upper arm) from the shoulder and are classified as either anterior or posterior. Anterior is by far the most common at a ratio of 10:1. Fractures of the head, or top part, of the humerus may be associated with dislocations. A replacement (reduction) of the dislocation should be attempted as soon as possible. Muscle spasm and pain will continue to increase the longer the dislocation is allowed to remain untreated.

Anterior dislocations may be identified by comparison to the opposite side. The normal smooth rounded contour of the shoulder, which is convex on the lateral (outside) side, is lost. With anterior displacement the lateral contour is sharply rectangular and the anterior (or front) contour is unusually prominent. The arm is held away from the body and any attempted movement will cause considerable pain. See Figure 4–6

A numb area located at the insertion of the deltoid muscle means that the axillary nerve has been damaged. Numbness or tingling of the little finger could mean ulnar nerve damage, while decreased sensation to the thumb, index, and middle finger may mean the radial nerve is injured. These findings increase the urgency of attempting a reduction.

The best method of reducing the anterior dislocation of the shoulder is the Stimson Maneuver. While other methods exist, this technique puts less force on the shoulder, which is particularly important in case fractures of the head of the humerus co-exist with the dislocation. The technique is illustrated in Figure 4–7. After reduction has been obtained, the arm is placed in a sling and a swathe is wrapped around the arm and chest to hold the arm against the body for three weeks. Mobilization too soon after reduction will result in a weak, unstable shoulder. In a young person this sling and swathe may be maintained for 4 weeks prior to range-of-motion exercise. Holding the position longer than 4 weeks will not reduce the chance of recurrent dislocation, while holding it there longer may result in a frozen shoulder.

Shoulder Blade

Fractures of the shoulder blade (scapula) are generally due to major trauma and the patient may require treatment for multiple fractures of the ribs, punctured lung (pneumothorax), or heart contusion. A direct blow to the scapula may fracture it without these other injuries. Diagnosis is difficult without an x-ray, but suspicion may be high if there is point tenderness to palpation over the scapula, particularly several days after the accident. An indication of scapular fracture is Comolli's Sign, which is a triangular swelling corresponding to the outline of the scapula. Treatment is with a sling and early mobilization to prevent stiffening of the shoulder.

Upper Arm Fractures (Near the Shoulder)

The humerus is the upper bone of the arm. Fractures of the upper part (or head) of the humerus are most common in elderly people. Again, the shoulder will be very painful. The classification of these fractures is made with x-rays, which would indicate that not only has a fracture occurred, but the number of pieces of the fracture and whether angulation or displacement has transpired. Displacement or severe angulation frequently requires surgical repair, but often very conservative measures are followed by the orthopedic specialist. Without access to x-ray or

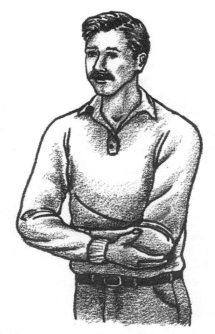

Figure 4-5:

A person with an anterior shoulder dislocation holds the arm away from the body and across the chest. Note the steep shoulder contour.

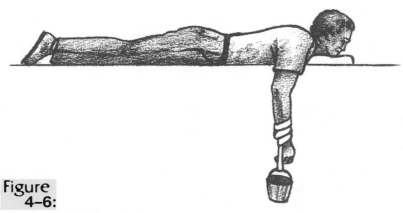

Figure 4-6:

The Stimson Method of replacing a dislocated shoulder. Using a wide cloth, wrap the forearm several times. Attach this wrap to a bucket or bag filled with 10 to 15 pounds of rocks and allow gravity to do the rest. It will take 20 minutes.

an orthopedic specialist we will have to treat all injuries conservatively.

Fractures of the upper humerus are associated with swelling and eventual bruising of the shoulder and upper arm, with gravity slowly causing the swelling and bruising to appear lower and lower down the arm. Severe pain will prevent normal movement of the shoulder, but some movement is frequently possible. As fractures of the upper part of the humerus occur through bone that mends itself readily (cancellous bone), the final outcome is often more dependent upon limiting the length of time of immobilization and starting proper physical therapy than it is upon the number of pieces or the separation and angulation. Conservative treatment will consist of a sling and swath (Figure 4–3). It is important in older individuals to mobilize the shoulder as soon as possible, otherwise adhesions form and a frozen shoulder results. An x-ray would help determine how much time should be allowed in the sling. This would range from only a few days to 4 or even 6 weeks with a four-part fracture with marked displacement. If the patient is over 30 the best rule of thumb while treating without x-ray is to mobilize and start physical therapy at 2 weeks. A youngster's arm can be left in a sling for 4 weeks. The therapy should consist of range-of-motion movements, such as circular elephant trunk motions while bending over, and raising the arm in front, to the side, and towards the rear. Effort should be made to move the shoulder as if the patient were wiping his bottom. The patient should do this on his own, without someone forcing his arm through these motions.

Upper Arm Fractures (Below the Shoulder)

Fractures beneath the head of the humerus—a region called "the neck"—will result in muscle spasm causing an over-riding of the shafts of bone. This is prevented by applying a hanging cast. This amounts to a weighted cast applied to the forearm with a loop of cloth supporting much of the weight of the cast from around the victim's neck. Mobilization and physical therapy should be started in two weeks. It is not practical in a setting without x-ray to properly design and follow the results of a hanging cast. Pain and apparent fracture of the humerus at the shoulder will probably have to be treated with a sling and swathe, with early mobilization as mentioned above.

Humeral shaft fractures take 2 to 4 months to heal. Located between the shoulder and the elbow, this is best splinted with a cast orthopedic surgeons call a "sugar tong" splint. It amounts to a U-shaped plaster extending from the armpit around the elbow back up to the shoulder, molded to the arm after reduction, and wrapped with an ace bandage. The Sam Splint can be used to construct a sugar tong splint, as in Figure 4–7.

Complete fractures of the shaft of the humerus will be very painful,

Figure 4-7: Legend: Sam Splint in sugar tong splint for humerus midshaft fracture.

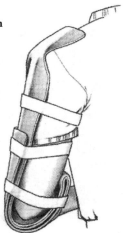

making a crunching feel when the bone is gently stressed. Incomplete fractures will be exquisitely tender to touch. Several days after the injury, swelling and bruising will appear at the elbow and forearm. Humeral shaft fractures at a point one-third of the way up from the elbow may cause damage to the radial nerve, thus causing numbness to the forearm, thumb, and index finger. This numbness generally lasts from 3 to 6 months and will commonly resolve on its own. Developing a numbness is a serious consequence that reflects either a tear or compression on a nerve. This is an area where the development of such a numb feeling is less cause for panic.

Elbow trauma

Fractures of the humerus above the elbow are very treacherous as bone fragments may seriously injure the nerves or blood vessels at this location. Fractures of the elbow itself are similarly dangerous due to the possible damage to nerve, blood vessel, or articular surfaces of the bones in this joint. The immense swelling associated with fractures or sprains at the elbow causes compression that frequently does more damage than sharp pieces of broken bone. Avoid splinting the elbow near a 90° angle. Allow the elbow to droop in the sling with a posterior padding. Never wrap the elbow joint at the front aspect—leave this area open to the air. It is compression in the front of the elbow joint, an area called the ante-cubital fossa, that frequently results in serious injury to the blood vessels and nerves. Surgical intervention with x-ray assistance is required to en-sure normal elbow function under many circumstances with regard to elbow fractures. Allowing the injured elbow to freeze into a 120° posi-tion may be the only treatment you can offer under long-term survival conditions.

Dislocation of the elbow is most common in young adults. Fractures of the tip of the elbow (the coronoid process) frequently are involved, but generally do not cause future problems. Fractures of the condyles can cause severe problems as indicated above, primarily due to compres-sion from associated bleeding on the neurovascular bundle. Reduction obviously should not be attempted if there is a chance of being treated properly by an orthopedic specialist with x-ray equipment. The appear-ance of the dislocated elbow would be obvious when compared to that person's other elbow. Some people have a sharper-looking elbow tip than the average individual. However, swelling and a particularly promi-nent, hard point behind the elbow would indicate that a dislocation has transpired.

Pain medication should be given to the victim to relax the muscles prior to attempting to reduce the dislocation. Figure 4–8 demonstrates the technique of reducing an elbow dislocation.

The ideal position after reduction of the elbow is at 90° with a posterior plaster splint. A 90° position is potentially dangerous as swelling may compromise the circulation. If the pulses at the wrist are decreased, then allow the elbow to droop as necessary to relieve this compression, possibly to a 120° position as described above. The reduction of a simple elbow dislocation is best maintained in the posterior splint for 3 weeks, then starting range-of-motion exercises. Soaking the elbow in warm water about 15 minutes prior to starting the gentle exercise program is helpful. If unusual deformity has resulted, or if the elbow is frozen, this frozen position may have to be accepted under survival conditions, until definitive surgery can be accomplished later. Full and proper use of this elbow will probably never again be established, even after the delayed surgery.

Forearm Fractures

Forearm fractures in children can generally be treated by reducing under x-ray and plaster casting, while in the adult they frequently are

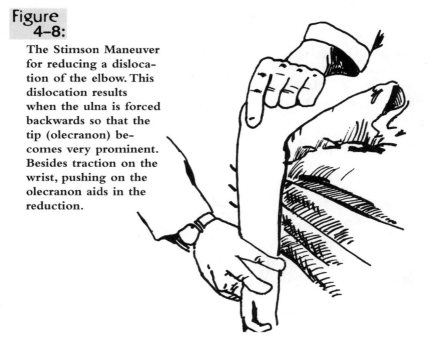

Figure 4–8:

The Stimson Maneuver for reducing a dislocation of the elbow. This dislocation results when the ulna is forced backwards so that the tip (olecranon) becomes very prominent. Besides traction on the wrist, pushing on the olecranon aids in the reduction.

treated surgically. Both options are not available to the isolated wilderness inhabitant if evacuation is not possible. The position of splinting of forearm fractures differs depending upon the location along the two bones, due to different forces upon these bones from tendon and muscle attachments. This positioning can only be held properly with tight-fitting plaster splints. Bone alignment can only be followed through repeated x-rays. Therefore it is obvious that a complete and unstable fracture of the forearm will very likely not heal properly when treated by crude techniques in a remote wilderness setting.

Most fractures of the forearm are not complete and unstable, however. They will heal nicely with protective splinting being the only required therapy. A stable crack can be suspected from swelling and point tenderness to gentle finger palpation by the examiner along the radius and ulna, the two forearm bones. Under this circumstance a splint must be manufactured that will provide stability so that this fracture can heal without danger of further trauma, as in Figure 4–9. The bone will weaken during the healing process and additional trauma may turn this non-displaced fracture into an angulated mess. Pad the splint well and provide a sling for at least 3 weeks. Keep splinted for a total of 6 weeks, longer if point tenderness is still present. If point tenderness disappears within a few days or at most 2 weeks, the injury was not a fracture, but simply a contusion, and the splint may be safely removed at that time.

Fractures associated with deformity in the forearm provide the physician with two challenges. First, reducing the fracture and second, maintaining its position with proper casting. Reduction of forearm fractures is generally done by traction, increasing the angulation to engage the fracture ends, then straightening the bones prior to casting. This is done

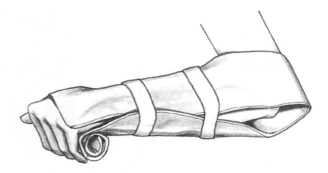

Figure 4–9:

Forearm splint technique with the Sam Splint.

with anesthesia. The survivalist had best splint deformed fractures of the forearm after straightening gross angulation with in-line traction. The splinted position will have to be maintained for 8 weeks or longer, depending upon the disappearance of local tenderness. A well-padded splint may generally be applied in a firm manner, immobilizing the elbow and wrist joints. Corrective surgery can be performed later. It is best to avoid a manipulation that will be extremely painful and unstable anyway.

Wrist Fractures and Dislocations

Wrist fractures and dislocations are common in young adults who extend their arms and hands to help break a fall. The three most common problems are fractures of the navicular (or scaphoid) bone, dislocation of the lunate, and perilunate dislocation. See wrist anatomy in Figure 4–10.

Navicular fractures frequently do not heal even with appropriate casting. Dislocations of the lunate or of the remaining carpals from the lunate would ideally be reduced, but without x-ray, experience, or at least local anesthesia this is not possible. Symptoms of lunate dislocation would be pain in the wrist and frequently numbness in the thumb, index, and middle fingers. There would be pain with any attempt to move the wrist. An abnormal nob on the palm side of the wrist at the crease, when compared to the other wrist, should be obvious to palpation. The numbness described indicates pressure on the median nerve from the dislocated navicular bone and an attempt at reduction

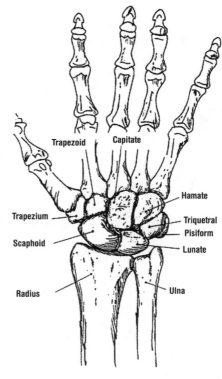

Figure 4–10: Anatomy of the wrist bones.

should be made. As in Figure 4–11, with the wrist in extreme dorsi-flexion, apply traction while attempting to push the lump back into position. The reduction often is accompanied by an obvious pop.

Perilunate dislocation will have similar symptoms and signs, with pain of attempted movement of the wrist and possible median nerve compression causing thumb, index finger, and middle finger numbness. The nob will not be present, but there will be a slight deformity of the back side of the wrist, sometimes called a modified silver fork deformity or hump at the upper side (dorsum) of the wrist. The technique of reduction is similar; apply traction to the wrist and place your thumb firmly over the location of the lunate bone (just beyond the end of the ulna) to hold the lunate in position as the wrist is then gradually flexed to bring the rest of the carpal bones down into proper position with the lunate and the ends of the radius and ulna. There is generally no snap when this occurs. The numb feeling should wear off within the next hour if the pressure has been removed from the median nerve.

Navicular (scaphoid) fractures will have pain particularly on the thumb side of the wrist, and while the entire wrist will be sore to palpation, it will be particularly sore below the thumb at the wrist. This fracture seldom dislocates, but it often doesn't heal, even after being placed in a tight plaster cast for several months.

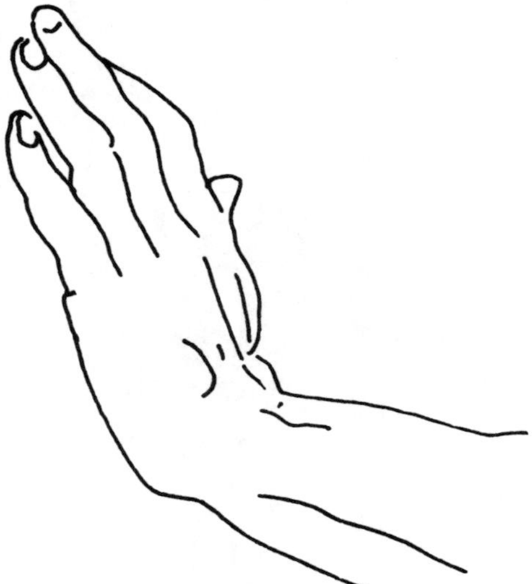

After attempting to reduce a dislocation of the wrist or treat the possible fracture of the navicular, splint the wrist and thumb so they are as immobile as possible. While it is not a rigid dressing, a thick wrap using a 2-inch ace applied in the manner called a *thumb spica* as illustrated in Figures 4–12 A and B can do fairly well. Under survival con-

Figure 4–11: Extreme dorsiflexion of the wrist. This is the position of the wrist used to aid in the reduction of the lunate bone dislocation.

ditions fusion, arthritis, even loss of median nerve function, may have to be accepted. This is a terrible loss that proper orthopedic treatment can almost always avoid. The thumb spica wrap will be adequate for sprains of the wrist and thumb.

Thumb Sprains and Fractures

Injuries causing severe pain and swelling of the thumb may be sprains or fractures. A severe sprain will cause loss of strength of the thumb for many weeks, even months. Swelling can be substantial with either injury. The first aid management is splinting until treatment by a physician can be arranged. In an extended survival situation, reduce any obvious deformity and hold in position with a thumb spica wrap, as in Figures 4–12 A and B. Severe sprains and all fractures will take 8 weeks to heal. There is risk of arthritis and loss of function depending upon the injury, patient's age, adequacy of reduction, and suitability of your splinting technique.

Hand Fractures

A hand fracture of the first metacarpal can be treated with a thumb spica wrap that immobilizes the entire wrist. The fifth metacarpal is the most commonly broken bone in the hand. The name given to this fracture, a "boxer's fracture," indicates its frequent method of origin. Perfect reduction of this fracture is not required, in fact up to 30 degrees of an-

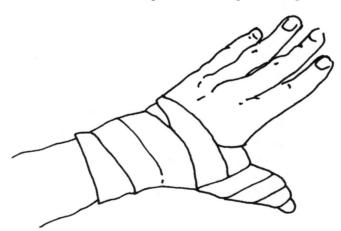

Figure 4-12: (A) The thumb spica wrap and (B) a thumb spica made with a Sam Splint.

gulation is acceptable. Only 5 to 10 degrees of angulation are acceptable in the third and fourth metacarpals. Measuring the amount of angulation will be impossible without an x-ray. If you are used to seeing these fractures, before and after x-rays become merely a legal maneuver and are not medically necessary. In the survival situation one may be able to tell if too much angulation has occurred by palpating the palm of the hand. If the nodular head of the metacarpal is felt where it joins the finger, there may be too much angulation. If too much angulation is allowed, a lump in the palm of the hand will make holding tools and objects uncomfortable for the rest of the patient's life. Splinting should be maintained in a position of function for 6 weeks. Unacceptable angulation will have to be snapped back into place.

Finger Fractures and Sprains

Gross lateral or sideways deviations of fingers should be corrected and the finger splinted in the position of function. These deviations may be corrected by tugging and thus resetting the fracture or by placing a pencil or similar object between fingers and thus getting leverage to snap a deviated finger shaft back into place. Deviations at the joints probably represent dislocations and these may be easily reduced by the tugging technique generally. An alternate technique to tugging is to place the dislocated joint into partial flexion; it will then be easier to lever the joint into position. Swelling associated with "jammed" fingers can become permanent if use of the finger is allowed before adequate healing has taken place. After the acute injury, splinting in the position of function is always appropriate for at least 3 weeks, followed by buddy splinting to the adjacent finger for another 2 to 3 weeks. Fingers should not be splinted straight. Buddy splinting may be used initially if the victim must use the hand immediately, as in canoeing, etc.

Ruptured tendons can be repaired generally by splinting in a position of function with the exception of a rupture of the distal extensor tendon of a finger. This injury is rather common and can be caused by an object hitting the tip of the finger or catching the finger in something (often in a sheet while making a bed). While making beds may not be a problem of the wilderness, this illustrates how easy the injury may occur. Figure 4–13 illustrates the appearance of this injury, commonly called a mallet finger deformity. The splinting technique for this injury is not the position of function, but as illustrated in Figure 4–14.

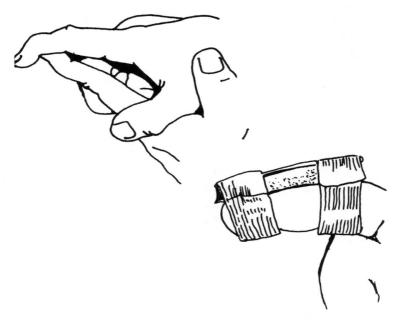

Figure 4–13: Mallet finger deformity from ruptured distal extensor tendon.

Figure 4–14: Splint technique for the ruptured distal extensor tendon.

Hip Dislocation and Fracture

Hip injuries are very serious. Tremendous blood loss occurs internally. Fractures of the hip cause pain in the anterior medial aspect (front and side) of the thigh. Dislocations in younger people may be associated with fractures; in older people fractures are very common and are the probable cause of the deformity. See Figure 4–15 A, B, and C for positions of fracture and dislocation.

Posterior dislocation of the hip is more common in healthy young adults compared to central fracture/dislocations and anterior hip dislocations. All these injuries are infrequent when compared, for instance, with dislocation of the shoulder. Posterior dislocations can cause injury to the sciatic nerve, the main nerve of the leg. This can cause shooting pains down the back of the leg and/or numbness of the lower leg. It is most important that reduction of the dislocation not be delayed longer than 24 hours. Muscle relaxation and pain medication must be given. To reduce, place the victim on her back with the knee and hip in a 90° position. The line of the femur should point vertically upwards. The thigh should be pulled steadily upwards while simultaneously rotating the femur externally, as shown in Figure 4–16.

For evacuation purposes, pad well and buddy splint to the other leg. This victim is a litter case. Continued pressure on, or severe injury to, the sciatic nerve will cause muscle wasting and loss of sensation to practically the whole leg. This damage must be surgically repaired as soon as possible, or in the extreme case of survival without possible repair, brace the affected leg to allow mobility by the victim and take care of numb skin areas to prevent sores and infection.

Central fracture/dislocations result when the head of the femur is driven through the socket into the pelvis. As in all orthopedic injuries an x-ray is almost essential for the diagnosis. If the fragments can be replaced surgically, this is the treatment of choice. In the extreme survival situation (such as no hope of medical care for many months), this injury can be left alone and still result in a stable and relatively painless joint. Light traction can be applied to the lower leg for comfort. After 3 weeks ambulation with crutches, gradually increasing weight can be encouraged. Range of motion exercises of the hip should be started from the beginning to help mold the healing fragments into a relatively smoother joint surface. Sciatic nerve injury should not occur with this injury, but an arthritic joint will result.

Anterior dislocation results from forceful injuries as in airplane crashes and motorcycle accidents. The examination of the lower leg demonstrates considerable lateral rotation or outward tilting of the foot when the victim is lying on his back. Reduction is as described under posterior dislocation with traction on the flexed limb, but combined with medial rotation, or rotating the limb inward rather than outward.

Thigh Fractures

Fractures of the thigh (femur) can, of course, occur from the hip to the knee. They are classified and treated by the orthopedic specialist differently according to the locations of the break.

The first aid treatment consists of treating for shock and immobilizing, initially using a traction splint. Start by providing pain relief with gentle hands on in-line traction. Then rig a "trucker's hitch" or, weather permitting, tape directly to the skin to form the traction splint as illustrated in Figure 4–17.

Traction splinting is initially required as spasms from the powerful

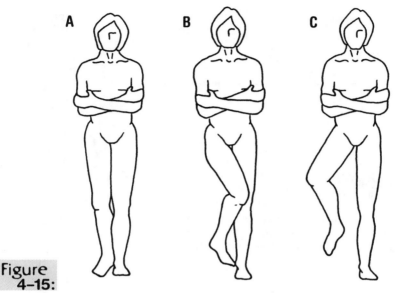

Figure 4-15:

(A) Typical appearance of a fractured hip; (B) typical appearance of a posterior hip dislocation; and (C) typical appearance of an anterior hip dislocation

muscles in this region cause considerable overriding of bone fragments, increasing the extent of the injury. Traction also re-establishes the normal length and configuration of the musculature and tightens the membranes that surround the muscle (the fascia), which very importantly decreases the bleeding that occurs with this injury. Additionally the application of a proper traction splint can result in significant pain reduction. During prolonged transport, it is possible that the patient can be comfortably removed from the traction splint periodically. After several days, he may do quite well with buddy splinting to the other leg during litter transport. Prolonged use of the trucker's hitch traction splint system can lead to necrosis, or death, to the skin of the ankle due to the constant pressure.

Knee Cap Dislocation

The knee cap (patella) usually dislocates laterally, or to the outside of the knee. This dislocation results in a locking of the knee with a bump to one side, making the diagnosis obvious. Relocate the patella by

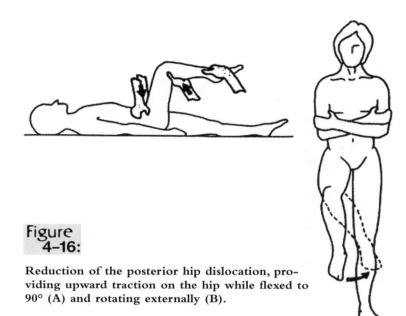

Figure 4-16:

Reduction of the posterior hip dislocation, providing upward traction on the hip while flexed to 90° (A) and rotating externally (B).

flexing the hip and the knee. When straightening the knee the patella usually snaps back into place by itself. If not, just push it back into place while straightening the knee on the next try. Splint with a tube splint (closed-cell foam sleeping pad), with the knee slightly flexed. This patient should be able to walk out.

Knee Sprains, Dislocations, or Fractures

The initial care of sprains, or acute joint injuries, is described on page 124. If the pain in the knee is severe, several diagnoses are possible. There may be tears of ligaments, tendon, cartilage, and/or synovial membranes. There may be associated dislocations or fractures. All you really can assess is the amount of pain that the patient is experiencing and you have to take his word for that. You can visually assess the amount of swelling or deformity and that might tell the tale, but the most important aspect of care will be handling pain as the patient interprets it.

Have the patient lie as comfortably as possible. Rest, Ice, Compress, and Elevate (RICE) the knee. In case of significant pain and/or swelling, remove the boot (weather permitting) and check the pulse on top of the foot (the dorsal pedal pulse); question the victim about sensation in the feet. Check the dorsal pedal pulse on the opposite side for comparison. If the injury appears minor, this is not necessary.

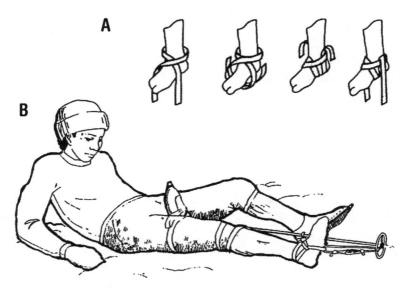

A

B

**Figure
4–17:**

(A) Apply webbing to form a trucker's hitch to prepare a traction splint in the field. (B) The trucker's hitch is attached to a ski pole padded with a shoe. This applies traction to the leg when pulled tight and tied off.

Significant deformity means that a dislocation may have occurred. Serious disruption of the blood vessels and nerve damage can occur. Check the pulses and check for sensation in the foot. If these are alright, splint the knee as it lies. If not, have a helper hold the lower thigh while you grip the ankle with one hand and the calf with the other. Use in-line traction while you gently flex the knee to see if you can reposition it better. If the pain is too great, you meet resistance, or you cannot do it, splint in the most comfortable position and evacuate as soon as possible.

Even without obvious deformity an immediate complaint, or continuing complaint, about significant pain means that you now have a litter case and you should make plans accordingly. If in two hours, the next morning, or two days later, the patient feels better and wishes to walk on it, great! Let her do it. You had best remove all weight from her shoulders and provide her with a cane. Have her use the cane on the side opposite the injury. This places a more natural force vector on the injured joint. And continue the compressive dressing. After two days begin applying heat packs during rest stops and in the evening. The patient's perception of pain should be the key to managing these injuries in the bush, although this approach can be complicated by varying pain thresholds, from macho to wimp.

Ankle Sprains, Dislocations, or Fractures

Generally fractures of both sides of the ankle are associated with a dislocation. The severe pain associated with the fractures will be an early indication that this patient is a litter case. Splint the ankle with a single Sam Splint or form a trough of ensolite foam and tape it on. The latter is not a walking splint, but if the pain is significant enough, the patient isn't walking anyway. A *flail* ankle, caused by complete disruption of the ankle ligaments, readily slops back into position and can be held in place with a trough splint of ensolite padding.

Allow the patient to rest after the injury before attempting to walk on the ankle. If there is severe pain, it might be broken or badly sprained. Either way, if the pain is too severe, the patient won't be walking. At least not until it quiets down. As with the knee, if the pain diminishes enough that the victim can walk, allow them to do so without equipment and with a cane.

Foot Injuries

Stubbed toes can be buddy splinted to provide pain relief. If they have been stubbed to the extent that they deviate at crazy angles sideways, they should be repositioned before buddy taping. Place a pencil (or a similar width object) on the side opposite the bend, and use it as a fulcrum to help snap the toe back into alignment. Blood under the toenail can be treated as described on page 114.

Severe pain in the arch of the foot or in the metatarsals can represent fractures or sprains. RICE as described above. Allowing a little time to lapse before use might result in decreasing pain in minor injuries, but it would take weeks for a fracture to decrease in severity. Decrease the patient's weightload and provide a cane. If the foot swells to the extent that the boot cannot be placed on the foot, consider cutting it along the sides and taping the boot circumferentially around the ankle to hold it on the foot. This provides support for the foot, ankle, and the patient's favorite outdoor retailer.

Chest Injuries

Broken ribs may develop after a blow to the chest. Even a severe cough or sneeze can also crack ribs! Broken ribs have point tenderness or exquisite pain with the lightest touch over the fracture site. The pain at this site will be reproduced by squeezing the rib cage in such a manner as to put a stress across the fracture site. Deep breathing will also produce pain at that location.

It is not necessary to strap or band the chest, except that such a band might prevent some rib movement and make the patient more comfortable. It is very important for the patient to breathe and have some cough reflex to aid in pulmonary hygiene, namely, to prevent the accumulation of fluid in the lungs, which can rapidly lead to pneumonia. Simply tying a large towel or undershirt around the victim's chest should suffice. A fractured rib will take 6 to 8 weeks to heal. A similar pain may be initially present due to a tear of the intercostal muscles or separation of cartilage from the bone of the rib near the sternum or breastbone. These problems are treated as above. They heal much quicker, generally three to five weeks.

If several adjacent ribs are broken in more than one location, a section of the chest wall is literally detached and held in place by the muscles and skin. This section of the chest wall can bulge out when the patient exhales instead of contracting as the chest would normally do. It can also move in when the rest of the chest expands during inhalation. This paradoxical motion of the chest wall is called a *flail chest*. Treatment includes placing an adequately sized rolled cloth against the flair portion to stabilize the motion. This cloth roll will have to be bound in place.

Treat all of the above conditions with pain medication as described on page 30. Avoid unnecessary movement. Have the patient hold his hand or a soft object against his chest when coughing to prevent rib movement and decrease the pain. Allow the patient to assume the most comfortable position, which is usually sitting up. If a fever starts, treat with antibiotic such as Levaquin 500 mg one daily.

Broken ribs usually heal well even though considerable movement seems to occur due to breathing or even flailing of the chest. They are always so painful that patients feel like they might puncture their lung at any minute. This does not usually happen, but if it does, there is a chance that air will leak into the chest cavity causing a pneumothorax. This can lead to significant respiratory distress to include cyanosis (blue discoloration of the skin due to inadequate oxygen in the blood). Crepitation can form in the skin. This is a crackling sensation that is very noticeable to the examiner when running the fingers over the skin in the upper part of the chest. It is not painful, but it indicates that air leakage and a pneumothorax has occurred. A pneumothorax can resolve on its own or it can expand, causing death. There is nothing that you can do for this unless you are trained in its management. Similarly, bleeding into lung tissue can result in a hemothorax, which can either resolve on its own or progress to death. Cyanosis, with difficult breathing, may also result due to this condition.

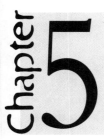

Chapter 5

Bites and Stings

Bee Stings

Stings from bees, wasps, yellow jackets, hornets (members of the *Hymenoptera* family), and fire ants produce lesions that hurt instantly and the pain lingers. The danger comes from the fact that some persons are "hypersensitive" to the venom and can go into immediate, life-threatening anaphylactic shock.

The pain of the sting can be alleviated by almost anything applied to the skin surface. Best choices are cold compresses, hydrocortisone 1% cream, or the triple antibiotic with pramoxine ointment from the Topical Bandaging Module. The use of oral pain medication such as Percogesic or stronger prescription pain medications can be given as necessary. Delayed swelling can be prevented and/or treated with oral antihistamines such as the diphenhydramine 25 mg taken 4 times daily from the Non-Rx Oral Medication Module. Sting relief is obtained with the application of the Sawyer Extractor (see page 158).

A generalized rash, asthmatic attack, or shock occurring within 2 hours of a sting indicates anaphylaxis, which requires special management.

Anaphylactic Shock

While most commonly due to insect stings, *anaphylactic shock* may result from a serious allergic reaction to medications, shellfish, and other foods, in fact to anything to which one has become profoundly allergic. Some nonstinging insect bites can also produce anaphylactic shock, for example, from the cone-nosed beetle (a member of the *Reduviidae* family) located in California and throughout Central and South America. We are not born sensitive to these things, but become allergic with repeated exposures. Those developing anaphylaxis generally have warnings of their severe sensitivity in the form of welts (urticaria) forming all over their body immediately after exposure, the development of an asthmatic attack with respiratory wheezing, or the onset of symptoms of shock.

While these symptoms normally develop within 2 hours and certainly before 12 hours, this deadly form of shock can begin within seconds of exposure. It cannot be treated as indicated in the section on "normal" shock on page 15. The antidote for anaphylactic shock is a prescription drug called epinephrine (Adrenalin). It is available for emergency use as a component of the Anakit (use is described on page 228) or in a special automatic injectable syringe called the EpiPen. See Figure 5–1. I recom-

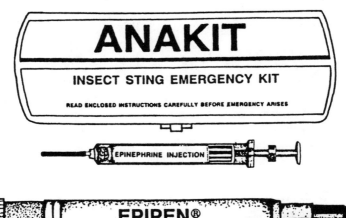

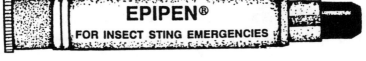

mend the Anakit as it contains two injections of epinephrine, rather
than one, and the cost is about half that of the EpiPen. Normal dose use
is 0.3 cc for an adult of the 1:1000 epinephrine solution given "subQ"
(in the fatty layer beneath the skin). While it is not necessary to treat the
itchy, generalized rash, the epinephrine should be given if the voice becomes husky (signifying swelling of the airway) and if wheezing or
shock occurs. This injection may have to be repeated in 15 to 20 minutes if the symptoms return. The Anakit contains a chewable antihistamine that should also be taken immediately, but antihistamines are of no
value in treating the shock or asthmatic component of anaphylaxis. Antihistamines can help prevent delayed allergic swelling and might be
somewhat protective from irregular heartbeats. If you have oral or injectable Decadron, give a 4 mg tablet or 4 mg injection for long-term
protection, which lasts over the next 12 hours.

A less expensive version of the Anakit is the AnaGuard, which consists
of only the syringe found in the Anakit, housed in a small protective
plastic case. This would provide you with 2 adult injections of epinephrine at a current retail cost of less than $24. Two EpiPens retail for $100.
The dose for persons under 12 years of age is one-half the adult dose,

which can be given by using the automatic injection EpiPen Jr or giving approximate amounts with the Anakit/AnaGuard syringe.

Evacuate anyone experiencing anaphylactic reactions even though they have responded to the epinephrine. They are at risk of the condition returning and they should be monitored carefully over the next 24 hours. People can die of anaphylaxis very quickly, even in spite of receiving aggressive medical support in a hospital emergency department. Beyond 24 hours they are no longer at risk of an anaphylactic reaction. If the patient is still alive after that time, vital signs are stable, and there is no manifestation of anaphylaxis, the evacuation can be terminated.

Snake Bite
Identifying Common North American Poisonous Snakes

With regard to the visual identification of the most common poisonous snakes in North America, pit vipers take their name from the deep pit, a heat receptor organ, between each eye and nostril. Most of them have triangular heads and cat-like vertical elliptical pupils. Further identifying information, including color photos, can be found at www.adventure-media.com/wilderness-medicine5/.

Coral snakes (*Micruruns fulvis,* Family Elapidae), while not pit vipers, also have vertical elliptical pupils. Some nonpoisonous snakes do as well. Color variations in coral snakes make the old saying that if "red-on-yellow can kill a fellow, red-on-black, venom lack" a very treacherous method of identification. This is particularly true in Central and South America. Coral snake bites should be treated as described under "Neurotoxic Snake Bites," below.

The essential steps in treating snake bites are: calm the victim, cause no additional harm, decide about evacuation urgency, and arrange for appropriate long-term wound care. The field first aid care of snake bites differs among nonpoisonous snakes, pit vipers (including rattle snakes, cottonmouth water moccasins, and copperheads—the family *Crotalidae*), and neurotoxic snakes (coral snakes, cobra, green mamba, krait, and all poisonous Australian snakes—the family *Elapidae*). That being said, the actual first aid care is easy to accomplish and will generally depend on where geographically the snake bite occurs. Treat North American pit viper snake bites without compression and treat snake bites received elsewhere as neurotoxic bites requiring compression and immobilization, as indicated below.

Regardless of the type of snake bite, the first step is to calm the patient and treat for shock. How do you calm a person who has just been bitten by a snake? Not surprisingly, just telling him to remain calm won't work. In a remote area when something terrible has happened, it's only your actions and demeanor that will provide comfort. Depending on the individual you may need to treat for shock immediately as described on page 16.

All snake bites are puncture wounds, and nonpoisonous bites and "dry" North American pit viper bites should be treated as indicated in the puncture wound section on page 102. Studies indicate that 20% of Eastern diamondback rattlesnake and 30% of cottonmouth water moccasin bites are dry, which means no venom has been injected into the victim.

Signs and Symptoms of Pit Viper Bite

What are the signs and symptoms of envenomation from these pit vipers? The first symptom noted by many is a peculiar tingling in the mouth, often associated with a rubbery or metallic taste. This symptom may develop in minutes and long before any swelling occurs at the bite site. Envenomation may produce instant burning pain. Weakness, sweating, nausea, and fainting may occur either with poisonous or nonpoisonous snake bites, due simply to the trauma of being bitten. In case of envenomation, within 1 hour there will generally be swelling, pain, tingling and/or numbness at the bite site. As several hours pass, bruising (ecchymosis) and discoloration of the skin begin and become progressively worse. Blisters may form, which are sometimes filled with blood. Chills and fever may begin, followed by muscle tremor, decrease in blood pressure, headache, blurred vision, and bulging eyes. The surface blood vessels may fill with blood clots (thromboses), and this can in turn lead to significant tissue damage after several days.

Treatment of Pit Viper Bite

For rattlesnakes, copperheads, and water moccasins (Family *Crotalidae*), treat for shock and calm the patient as indicated above. Immediately apply suction using a Sawyer Extractor to the puncture wound(s) without making any incisions. Rubber suction cups are worthless, as is mouth suction. Studies of the Sawyer Extractor show that application within 3 minutes of the bite can extract 35% of the venom. More rapid application might extract much more, but this has not been studied. After half an hour of application less than 3% additional venom will be removed so that further suction can be terminated. The immediate application of the Sawyer Extractor (see Figure 5–2) is safe, effective, and very reassuring to the victim, although you may need to show the patient that it is a vacuum device rather than one of the world's largest shots! Immobilize the injured part at heart level or slightly below. And evacuate if you can.

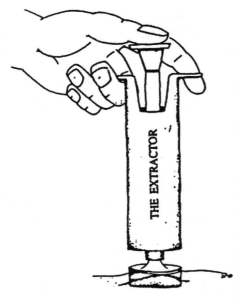

Figure 5–2: The Sawyer Extractor applies vacuum to a wound to treat snake and insect bites.

It has been said that the best snake bite kit is a set of car keys. The reason is that envenomation can make a person very ill (on average 7 people die yearly in North America from these bites), and it can cause serious tissue damage that is best treated with antivenin. There is a golden hour and a half before North American pit viper venom causes significant generalized effects that might make the victim nonambulatory. You might want to start walking the victim toward the nearest road to shorten the length of a litter evacuation, which will become necessary if his condition deteriorates. This walk-out should be performed in a calm, but urgent manner. Attempting to carry any but a very light individual will excessively prolong this trip out.

Do not apply compression or a tourniquet to the swelling associated with this type of bite because the venom causes considerable tissue damage from squeezing blood vessels and further compression makes this effect worse. Do not apply ice as this results in increased local tissue destruction. Avoid the use of a constricting band between the bite site and the heart as this has never been shown to be effective and there is a real danger of its been applied too tightly, resulting in a tourniquet effect that increases tissue destruction.

The antivenin available in North America, produced by Wyeth, is a polyvalent *Crotalidae* antivenin made from horse serum. It is effective against all species of North American pit vipers, therefore it is not necessary to identify the snake. The amount of antivenin given will depend upon the amount and rapidity of onset of swelling around the bite site. The exception to this is the Mojave Rattler, which has a virulent venom that does not cause the local signs of the other pit viper envenomation. Potential bites by this rattler are given aggressive amounts of antivenin. Many people are highly sensitive to the horse serum and for some of these people this antivenin preparation may be more lethal than the snake bite. The use of the Wyeth antivenin is not practical in the field and I would not suggest carrying it, even on snake gathering expeditions.

Neurotoxic Snake Bites

Coral snakes, and all Australian, most African, Indian, and South American snakes (most in Family *Elapidae*) are all capable of injecting neurotoxins into their victim's system with their bite. In 1979 Australia adapted pressure/immobilization as the first aid treatment for the very dangerous snakes found on that continent and dropped their yearly death rate from snake bite to virtually zero. The Sawyer Extractor is not used initially in Australia, but a friend used one in Africa on a mamba bite, pulling a large quantity of yellow fluid out prior to pressure/immobilization and is convinced that this saved the patient's life. Due to the availability of excellent, specific antivenins in Australia, pressure/immobilization and transporting negates the need for initial Sawyer Extractor use. In areas of the world where access or availability of antivenin may be doubtful, first use the Sawyer Extractor, if it can be applied immediately, and apply pressure/immobilization within 1 minute.

In Australia the wound is not washed prior to wrapping, as special "Venom Detection Kits" are available at hospitals that can identify the snake from venom in the wound. The wound is not manipulated in any way; instead, pressure/immobilization is applied immediately as indicated in Figure 5–3. Sawyer of Australia produces a pressure/immobilization snake bite kit that is available over the Internet from Main Peak in Perth (www.iinet.net.au/~mainpeak/).

Treatment of Coral Snake Bite

North American coral snakes envenomate by a slow chewing process, so that a rapid withdrawal from the attack may result in no envenomation. For treatment: (1) Treat for shock as necessary; (2) wash the bitten area promptly to possibly remove some venom; (3) apply suction with the Sawyer Extractor; (4) make no incisions; (5) apply pressure/immobilization; (6) evacuate to a hospital if possible.

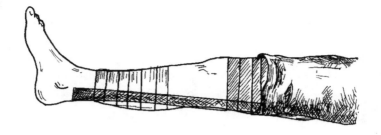

Figure 5-3:

How to apply pressure/immobilization for neurotoxic snake bites:

(A) Apply a broad pressure bandage over the bite site as soon as possible. Do not take off clothing as any movement helps the venom to enter the blood stream.

(B) The elastic bandage should be as tight as you would apply to a sprained ankle.

(C) Extend the bandage as high as possible, wrapping over clothing if necessary.

(D) Apply a splint to the leg.

(E) Bind the splint to as much of the leg as possible.

(F) Bites on hand or forearm: 1. Bind to elbow with bandage. 2. Splint to elbow. 3. Use sling. *(Adapted from* Venomous Creatures of Australia, *Oxford University Press, copyright 1994 Struan Sutherland, used with permission.)*

Since the coral snake is an elapid, like the cobra, signs and symptoms of envenomation take time to develop and deterioration then proceeds so rapidly that the antidote may be of no avail. Many experts feel the antidote should be given immediately after skin testing in all cases. Most authorities feel 2 units of the Wyeth Micruris fulvis antivenin should be given intravenously immediately at the hospital. Some use 10 amps of the antivenin. Made from horse serum, this antivenin is not suitable for field use.

Cobra, Russell's viper, green mamba, and krait bites outside of Australia result in thousands of deaths yearly. While many areas of the world have a local source of antivenin for the species of snakes that are of concern in that locale, often the antivenin may be inaccessible. The use of a class of compounds called anticholinesterases can be life-saving when dealing with neurotoxic envenomations when no antivenin is available. For physician use only, a suggested protocol is the administration of .6 mg of atropine IV (.05 mg/kg for children) to control intestinal cramping followed by 10 mg of Tensilon (0.25 mg/kg for children). If there is improvement, further control of symptoms can be obtained by titration of a dose of neostigmine 0.025 mg/kg/hr by IV injection or continuous infusion. These medications are *not* included in the recommended Rx Injectable Module.

Insect Bites and Stings

Spider Bites

Generally spiders will make a solitary bite, not several. If you wake with multiple bites, you have probably collided with some other arthropod. While only some spiders are considered poisonous, all spiders have venom that can cause local tissue inflammation and even slight necrosis or destruction. Most spiders are unable to bite well enough to inject the venom.

Black Widow Spider

The black widow *(Latrodectus mactans)* is generally a glossy black with a red hourglass mark on the abdomen. Sometimes the hourglass mark is merely a red dot, the two parts of the hourglass do not connect, or the coat is not shiny and it may contain white. (A color photograph of this spider can be seen on my Web site. The bite may only be a pin-prick, but generally a dull cramping pain begins at the site within 15 minutes, which may spread gradually until it involves the entire body. The muscles may go into spasms and the abdomen becomes board-like. Extreme restlessness is typical. The pain can be excruciating. Nausea, vomiting, swelling of eyelids, weakness, anxiety (naturally), pain on breathing may all develop. A healthy adult can usually survive, with the pain abating in several hours and the remaining symptoms disappearing in several days.

An ice cube on the bite, if available, may reduce local pain. A specific antidote is available (*L. mactans* antivenin from Merck & Company), which should be given (after skin testing) to persons under 16 and over 65, heart or kidney patients, or those with very severe symptoms. The dose is one vial diluted in 15 to 50 ml of saline and given intravenously over 10 minutes. A specific treatment for relieving muscle spasm is methocarbamol (Robaxin) 100 mg given as a bolus into an IV line at 1 ml/min. After the initial bolus, a constant infusion of 200 mg/hr IV or 500 mg by mouth every 6 hours can be used. This medication has not been included in the Wilderness Medical Kit, but adequate pain relief can be given by using Percogesic from the Non-Rx Oral Medication Module, or the Lorcet 10/650.

Similar spiders are found throughout the world. The South African knoppie, the New Zealand katipo, and the Australian red black spider bites have the same symptoms and can all be treated as described above. A specific antivenin is available in those countries.

Brown Recluse Spider

A brown coat with a black violin marking on the cephalothorax or top part identifies the brown recluse spider *(Loxosceles reclusa)*. (A color photograph of this spider can be seen on my Web site. The initial bite is mild and may be overlooked at the time. In an hour or two, a slight redness may appear; by several hours a small bleb appears at the bite site. Sometimes the wound appears as a bull's eye with several rings of red and blanched circles around the bite. The bleb ruptures, forming a crust, which then sloughs off; a large necrotic ulcer forms, gradually enlarging. Over the first 36 hours, vomiting, fever, skin rash, and joint pain may develop and hemolysis of the blood may be massive.

Apply ice to the wound as soon as possible. An antivenin has been developed from rabbits and is being used experimentally. Dapsone 100 mg twice daily (a medication used in the treatment of leprosy) has been used, but its effectiveness has been questioned. Dapsone, once thought to be effective during the early stages of treatment to decrease the severity of the inflammation, is not included as a routine component of the

Wilderness Medical Kit. Prophylactic use of antibiotics does no good. Avoid the application of heat to this wound, even though it is inflamed and necrotic.

Give ibuprofen 200 mg 4 tablets every 6 hours to help with pain and to reduce inflammation. From the Rx Oral/Topical Module give Decadron 4 mg every 6 hours. (Your medical kit supply will be exhausted in 2½ days, but it is doubtful that steroid therapy is of benefit after that time.) Apply triple antibiotic ointment from the Topical Bandaging Module and cover with Spenco 2nd Skin dressing.

Ticks

More vector-borne diseases are transmitted in the United States by ticks than by any other agent (see Table 6–1). Ticks must have blood meals to survive their various transformations. It is during these meals that disease can be transmitted to humans and other animals. Two families of ticks can transmit disease to humans: the *Ixodidae,* or hard ticks, and the *Argasidae,* or soft ticks. The life cycle of the hard tick takes 2 years to complete: from the egg, the six-legged larva or seed tick, the eight-legged immature nymph, and the eight-legged mature adult. They must remain attached for hours to days while obtaining their blood meal. Disease will not be transferred if the tick can be removed before 24 hours. Pictures of the North American *Ixodidae* with maps of the distribution of these ticks are located at my Web site. The soft ticks can live many years without food. They have several nymphal stages and may take multiple blood meals. They usually stay attached less than 30 minutes. Of the soft ticks, only the genus *ornithodoros* transmit disease in the United States, namely, relapsing fever. The 24 hour rule does not apply in this case.

Prevention of attachment is the best defense against tick-borne disease. DEET insect repellents are very effective against ticks (see page 164). Permethrin 0.5% spray-treated clothing kills ticks upon contact and remains active on clothing for 2 weeks. Then it's probably about time to wash those camping clothes anyway and re-spray them. The combination of permethrin on clothing and DEET on skin is 100% effective against tick attachment.

OK, so you didn't follow my advice and you find a tick attached. How do you remove it? A tried-and-true method is to grasp the skin around the insertion of the tick with a pair of fine point tweezers, and pull straight outward, removing the tick and a chunk of skin. For some reason this doesn't hurt. A recent study has shown the effectiveness of three products on the market in the United States sold under the brand names of The Original Ticker Off, The Pro-Tick Remedy, and the Tick Plier, which is also sold under the name the Tick Nipper.★ Hot wires, matches, glue, fingernail polish, Vaseline, none of them work. Burning the tick might cause it to vomit germs right into the victim, yet it will not let go. Be careful not to grasp the tick body—crushing it might also cause germs to be injected into the victim.

Caterpillar Reactions

The puss caterpillar (*Megalopyge opercularis*) of the southern U.S. and the gypsy moth caterpillar (*Lymantria dispar*) of the Northeast have bristles that cause an almost immediate skin rash and welt formation. Treatment includes patting the victim with a piece of adhesive tape to remove these bristles. Further treatment is discussed on page 116.

Millipede Reactions

Millipedes do not bite, but contact can cause skin irritation. Cold packs can reduce discomfort. Wash thoroughly and treat as indicated on page 116.

Centipede Bites

Some of the larger centipedes can inflict a painful bite that causes a local swelling and painful, red lesion. Treatment with a cold pack is usually sufficient. Some bites are severe and regional lymph node enlargement may occur, which will be a swelling of the nodes generally at the joints along the blood flow pattern towards the heart from the bite site. Swelling at the bite location may persist for weeks. Adequate treatment consists of pain medication. Infiltration of the area with lidocaine 1% from the Rx Injectable Module provides instant relief and is justified in severe cases.

Mosquitos

The best mosquito repellent invented to date has been DEET (n,n diethyl-m-toluamide). This product has undergone a revolution in the past 20 years, ranging from the earliest preparations of 12% strength to numerous products marketing 100% DEET concentration. Between 10 and 15% of DEET applied to the skin surface is excreted in the user's

★Stewart R.L., Burgdorfer W., and Needham G.R. Evaluation of three commercial tick removal tools. *Wilderness and Environmental Medicine* 1998; 9:137–142.

urine. This fact, coupled with a few reports of convulsions in children using DEET, indicates that we should probably minimize the total amount placed on the skin.

Two new formulations are being made to provide the effectiveness of a strong DEET concentration using lower amounts that are less readily absorbed. One is the use of a microencapsulate formula that keeps the DEET from being absorbed into the skin; this is being sold as Sawyer Controlled Release Insect Repellent. The other is the composite-based formula system that adds a synergist to enhance the effectiveness of lower concentrations of DEET. Probably the best product on the market at this time is a composite called Sawyer Gold, also made by Sawyer Products (P.O. Box 188, Safety Harbor, FL 34695). It consists of 17.5% DEET, 5% synergist N-octyl bicycloheptene dicarboximide (MGK 264, Synergist), and a black fly repellent, 2% Di-n-propyl Isocinchomeronate (MGK Repellent 326). A thin coating of Sawyer Gold lotion will last for many hours, even under tropical or Arctic conditions. I have used this product during enormous mosquito and black fly exposures and find that it works 6 to 12 hours. This minimizes the number of reapplications and the total DEET exposure tremendously.

I never use 100% DEET except to soak either my head netting or a "bug jacket." Bug jackets are a very loose weave of cotton fabric that soaks up DEET. The loose weave allows air circulation, which is a real life-saver during those hot mosquito-laden summer days. Buy one with a hood. Avoid buying the tight "no-see-um proof" mosquito suits, as you can sweat to death in them. Even during monstrous mosquito moments, it is possible to be relatively comfortable in a treated bug jacket. The hood can be pulled over your head when you are eating and your cup or bowl brought very near your face so that you can gulp down food that is relatively free of mired insects (except for those that fall into the pot during the cooking process). Treat the bug jacket by pouring 100% DEET into a zip-lock plastic bag and soaking the jacket overnight. The best brand of bug jacket I have found is the Ben's brand. Rather than wearing the tight weave net pants, I find it best to treat my trousers with permethrin, as indicated below, and my ankles or exposed legs with the DEET composite or delayed release formula as described above.

Adequate mosquito netting for the head and for the tent or cot while sleeping is essential. Spraying netting and clothing with .5% permethrin increases the effectiveness of the netting and decreases bug bites enormously. Permethrin is an insecticide, not a repellent. It kills mosquitos, ticks, black flies, etc., and does not simply chase them away. It will not work if applied to the skin, as an enzyme in the skin destroys it. Not only is there no absorption through the skin, it is safe to use on both natural and synthetic fibers.

I have not found vitamin B^1 (thiamine) to be an effective preventative oral agent, but the recommended dose by those who do is 100 mg daily for 1 week prior to departure and daily thereafter. Electronic sound devices to repel these critters have never dented mosquito buzzing or biting enthusiasm in the far north in my experience, but I have friends who use them enthusiastically (under less obnoxious circumstances).

A considerable number of bites, or sensitivity to bites, may require an antihistamine, such as diphenhydramine 25 mg capsules every 6 hours from the Non-Rx Oral Medication Module. Triple antibiotic ointment with pramoxine applied every 6 hours can provide local itch relief. Or from the Rx Oral/Topical Module use Topicort 2.5% ointment twice daily.

Black Flies

DEET compounds will work on black flies, but the concentration must be 30% or greater and even the pure formula will work only a short time. It is best to use a specific black fly repellent or a composite formula such as the Sawyer Gold, mentioned in the section on mosquitos.

For years Skin So Soft, a bath oil marketed by your local Avon representative, has been mentioned as a black fly repellent. It does work, but it requires frequent applications, approximately every 15 minutes.

Netting and heavy clothes that can be sealed at the cuffs may be required. All black fly species like to land and crawl, worming their way under and through protective clothing and netting. Spray clothing and netting with .5% permethrin as mentioned in the section on mosquitos.

Black fly bites can result in nasty sores that are usually self-limited, although at times slow healing. If infection is obvious, treat as indicated in the section on skin infection on page 116. Treat symptoms as indicated under mosquitos above.

No-See-Ums and Biting Gnats

These two examples of insect life are the scourge of the North Country, or any country in which they may be found. Many local people refer to any small black fly as a "no-see-Um," but the true bug by that name is indeed very hard to see. They usually come out on a hot, sticky night. The attack is sudden and feels like fire over your entire exposed body surface area. Under the careful examination of a flashlight, you will notice an incredibly small gnat struggling with its head down, merrily chomping away. Make that bug portion of the previous sentence plural please. This is an ideal time for application of the Sawyer Gold or you will have to resort to strong DEET product of 35% or greater. Immersion in cold water will help relieve symptoms temporarily. One remedy for the sting which I understand works quite well, but which I have never had along to try, is an application of Absorbine Jr!

Gnats, on the other hand, are small black flies whose bite is seldom felt. But these gentle biters leave behind a red pimple-like lesion to remind you of their visit. A rash of these pimples around the neck and ankles attests to their ability to sneak through protective clothing. Treat bites as described under mosquitos above. Without a head net or treated hooded bug jacket, hoards of gnats can suffocate you. Treat clothing with permethrin and the bug jacket with 100% DEET as described in the section about mosquitos.

Scorpion Sting

Most North American scorpion stings are relatively harmless. Stings usually cause only localized pain and slight swelling. The wound may feel numb. Diphenhydramine 25 mg 4 times daily and Percogesic 2 tablets every 4 hours may be all that is required for treatment. A cold pack will help relieve local pain.

The potentially lethal *Centruroides sculptuatus* is the exception to this rule. This yellow-colored scorpion lives in Mexico, New Mexico, Arizona, and the California side of the Colorado River. (A color picture of this scorpion is located on my Web site.) The sting causes immediate, severe pain with swelling and subsequent numbness. The neurotoxin injected with this bite may cause respiratory failure. Respiratory assistance may be required (see page 19). Tapping the wound lightly with your finger will cause the patient to withdraw due to severe pain. This is an unusual reaction and does not occur with most insect stings. A specific antivenin is available in Mexico and is also produced by the Poisonous Animals Laboratory at Arizona State University for local use. In addition to the antivenin, atropine may be needed to reduce muscle cramping, blurred vision, hypertension, respiratory difficulty, and excessive salivation. Methocarbamol may be given as described in the section on black widow spider bites (page 161). Neither of these medications are included in the Wilderness Medical Kit. Narcotics such as Demerol and morphine can increase the toxicity and should be avoided. Percogesic from the Non-Rx Oral Medical Module may be safely given.

Ant, Fire Ant

While many ants can alert you to their presence with a burning bite, fire ants can produce an intensely painful bite that pales any other ant—and many other bug—bite to insignificance. While holding on tightly with his biting pincer and pivoting around, the fire ant stings repeatedly in as many places as the stinger can reach, causing a cluster of small, painful blisters to appear. These can take 8 to 10 days to heal. Treatment is with cold packs and pain medication. Large local reactions may require antihistamine such as the diphenhydramine 25 mg, 2 capsules every 6 hours and even Decadron 4 mg twice daily. Local application of Spenco 2nd Skin can provide some relief. Treat with pain medication as required.

The greatest danger is to the hypersensitive individual who may go into *anaphylactic shock,* page 154.

Aquatic Stings

Sea Urchin

Punctures from sea urchin spines cause severe pain and burning. Besides trauma from the sharp spines, some species inject a venom. The wound can appear red and swollen or even blue to black from a harmless dye that may be contained in the spines. Generalized symptoms are rare, but may include weakness, numbness, muscle cramps, nausea, and occasionally shortness of breath. The spines should be removed thoroughly, a very tedious process. Very thin spines may be absorbed by the body without harm, but some may form a reactive tissue around them (granulomas) several months later. Spines may migrate into joints and cause pain and inhibit movement or lodge against a nerve and cause extreme pain. The discoloration of the dye causes no problems, but may be mistaken for a thin spine. Relief may be obtained by soaking in hot water (110 to 113° F or 43 to 45° C) for 20 to 30 minutes. Vinegar or acetic acid soaks several times a day may help dissolve spines that are not found. Evacuation and treatment by a physician is advisable.

Jellyfish

There is an extensive number of species of jellyfish in the world posing varying degrees of danger to people. Jellyfish tentacles in contact with human skin can cause mild pricking to burning, shooting, terrible pain. The worse danger is shock and drowning.

Pouring vinegar on the wound (4 to 6% acetic acid) inhibits the venom from being fired into the skin. Alcohol (or ideally formalin) poured over the wound, may also prevent the nematocysts from firing more poison. Avoid the use of hot water in treating this injury as water of *any* temperature activates the nematocysts. Try to remove the tentacles with gloved hands.

Powder the area with a dry powder such as flour or baking powder. Gently scrape off the mess with a knife, clam shell, or other sharp instrument, but avoid cutting the nematocysts with a sharp blade. Apply hydrocortisone 1% cream 4 times daily from the Topical Bandaging Module or Topicort 0.25% ointment twice daily from the Rx Oral/Topical Module for inflammation. Severe stings can be treated with pressure/immobilization. Provide rescue breathing as required.

Coral Stings

These injuries are treated as indicated under *jellyfish*.

Coral Cuts, Barnacle Cuts

Clean the wound thoroughly. Trivial wounds can later flare into real disasters that may go on for years. Scour thoroughly with a coarse cloth or soft brush and surgical scrub or soapy water. Then apply hydrogen peroxide to help bubble out fine particles and bacteria. Apply triple antibiotic ointment from the Topical Bandaging Module. Manage this wound as discussed in the section on laceration care, page 91. If an infection ensues, treat as indicated on page 116.

Sting Ray

The damage is done by the barbed tail, which lacerates the skin, imbedding pieces of tail material and venom into the wound. The wound bleeds heavily, pain increases over 90 minutes and takes 6 to 48 hours to abate.

Immediately rinse the wound with seawater and remove any particles of the tail sheath, which are visible as these particles continue to release venom. Hot water is the treatment of choice—applied as soon as possible and as hot as the patient can stand it (110 to 113° F, 43 or 45° C). The heat will destroy the toxin rapidly and remove the pain that the pa-

tient is experiencing. After hot water has been applied and all tail particles removed, the wound may be closed with taping techniques (see
page 95). Elevation of the wound is important. If particularly dirty, leave
the wound open and continue to use intermittent hot soaks as described
on page 115. Questionably dirty wounds should be treated with Levaquin 500 mg daily or doxycycline 100 mg twice daily from the Rx
Oral/Topical Medication Module. As these are nasty, painful wounds,
treat for shock from the onset.

Catfish

Apply hot water as indicated under *sting ray*. The wound must be
properly cleaned and irrigated using surgical scrub, if available, or soap.
Place the patient on oral antibiotics for several days to decrease the
chance of wound infection, which is common with this injury. Treat infected wound as described on page 116.

Scorpion Fish

Same treatment as *sting ray*.

Sponge Rash

Sponges handled directly from the ocean can cause an allergic reaction that appears immediately. Fine spicules may also break off in the
outer layer of skin causing inflammation. It will be difficult to tell
whether your victim is suffering from the allergic reaction or the
spicules, or both. Soak the affected skin by applying vinegar to a cloth
and covering for 15 minutes. Dry the skin and pat with the adhesive
side of tape to remove sponge spicules. Again soak in vinegar for 5 minutes. An application of rubbing alcohol for 1 minute has been suggested.
Then apply hydrocortisone 1% cream 4 times a day from the Topical
Bandaging Module or Topicort 0.25% ointment twice daily from the
Rx Oral/Topical Medication Module for several days until the inflammation subsides.

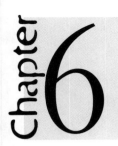

Chapter

6

Infectious Disease

The major concerns the outdoor and adventure traveler faces with regard to infectious diseases include their geographical distribution, the vector or method of transmission, the ability to prevent by lifestyle or immunization, and the availability of treatment. This book emphasizes North American illness and the most likely contagions to afflict adventure travelers while in developing countries. In some of these locations, many services, legal as well as medical, are actually deteriorating. Prior to any trip out of the country call the U.S. Department of State Advisory Hotline (202) 647–5225 for the latest information concerning political unrest. This number includes health issues at times. Also call the Centers for Disease Control and Prevention International Traveler's Hotline at (404) 332–4559. Links to the above organizations' Web sites, and other travel related information, will be found at www.adventure-media.com/travel/

The following tables summarize wilderness-related diseases found in North America and high-risk illnesses encountered in world travel.

Diseases of North America*

Table 6-1

Illness	Mode	Page Number
Babesiosis	tick	172
Blastomycosis	soil	173
Coccidiodomycosis	soil	174
Colorado Tick Fever	tick	174
Echinococcus	water	175
Ehrlichiosis	tick	176
Encephalitis	mosquito	176
Giardiasis	water	177
Hantavirus	rodents/soil	178

con't next page

Babesiosis

First discovered in Yugoslavia in 1957 and the United States in 1968, this is a malaria-like illness caused by a protozoan parasite that invades red blood cells. Two species have been identified, *Babesia microti* causing disease in the northeastern United States and *B. equi* causing disease in California. An unidentified species caused this disease in a patient in

Washington state. Over 450 confirmed cases have been reported from the offshore islands of the Northeast, Maryland, Virginia, Georgia, Wisconsin, Minnesota, California, and Washington. Several species of ixodes ticks transmit babesiosis. A map of the reported location of ixodes tick in North America is located on the Web site at www.adventure-media.com/wilderness-medicine5/.

Symptoms gradually begin 1 week after a tick bite with fatigue and loss of appetite, giving way in several days to fever, drenching sweats, muscle ache, and headache. The illness ranges from mild to severe, with death occurring in about 10% of patients. Treatment is available with oral quinine plus clindamycin (not included in the recommended medical kit). Protection from tick bites is best accomplished by treating clothing with permethrin (see page 163).

Blastomycosis

This infectious disease is caused by a fungus, *Blastomyces dermatitidis*. Outbreaks usually cluster with multiple members of a party becoming ill. It is found in the Mississippi River Valley and the southeastern United States. It is also found in various parts of Africa. In the United States it has been associated with beaver lodges and from digging in contaminated soil. It can also result from dog bites.

Onset of illness is slowly progressive, usually starting with a cough and developing into a pneumonia with fevers, shortness of breath, chest pain, and drenching sweats. Infected blood carries the fungus to the skin and other tissues. Skin lesions enlarge with a collapsed center, purplish-red border, and frequent ulcerations.

Antifungal drugs are available, such as oral ketoconazole, 800 mg given daily (not included in the recommended medical kit). In most untreated patients the disease is slowly progressive and fatal.

Cholera

This intestinal infection, caused by a bacterium *Vibrio cholerae,* produces profuse, cramping diarrhea. Death can come from dehydration; indeed, the death toll can reach the tens of thousands during an epidemic. Ingestion of water contaminated with the bacterium spreads the disease. Humans are the only documented hosts for this disease. In the past 20 years cholera has spread from India and Southeast Asia to Africa, the Middle East, and Southern Europe. Since 1991 thousands of cases have been reported in Peru and many other countries of South and Central America and Mexico. The current vaccine provides such low immunity that its use is not justified. No country officially requires cholera vaccine for entry. Check for latest information on active disease areas and countries requiring immunization for entry by contacting the International Association of Medical Assistance for Travellers (IAMAT) (see Appendix B).

The most important treatment is to use oral rehydration as indicated on page 82. The strain of cholera now raging in most of the world is very resistant to antibiotics and, fortunately, does not require antibiotic treatment. Imodium 2 mg can be used for symptomatic relief, 2 capsules immediately, with an additional capsule after each loose stool.

Coccidioidomycosis

Also called San Joaquin Fever or Valley Fever, coccidioidomycosis is a fungal infection caused by *Coccidiodes immitis*. Found in the San Joaquin Valley and throughout the southwestern United States, this disease is caught by inhaling the fungal spore in dust.

Symptoms can be delayed in travelers until after leaving the endemic area. The primary symptoms are those of an upper respiratory infection, bronchitis, or a pneumonia. Incubation time is varied and a progressive form may occur weeks, months, or years after the original infection in people with decreased immunity (AIDS patients, people on steroids, or those receiving chemotherapy).

Treatment is not required for those with upper respiratory infection symptoms. The diagnosis should be made with special blood tests to avoid missing other treatable pneumonia. Progressive disease must be treated with intravenous antifungal medications.

Colorado Tick Fever

A viral disease spread by *Ixodid* (hard-shelled) ticks, this disease is 20 times more common than Rocky Mountain spotted fever in Colorado. It is also found in the other states of the Western Rocky Mountains and provinces of Western Canada. It is most frequent in April and May at low altitudes and June through July at high altitudes.

Onset is abrupt, with chills, fever of 100.4° to 104° F (38° to 40° C), muscle ache, headache, eye pain, and eye sensitivity to light (photophobia). The patient feels weak and nauseated, but vomiting is unusual. During the first 2 days, up to 12% of the victims develop a rash. In half the cases the fever disappears after 2 to 3 days and the patient feels well for 2 days. Then a second bout of illness starts that lasts intensely for 2 to 4 days. This second phase subsides with the patient feeling weak for 1 to 2 additional weeks.

This disease requires no treatment other than bed rest, fluids to prevent dehydration, and medications to treat fever and aches. However, as the same ticks can also spread potentially dangerous Rocky Mountain spotted fever, treatment with doxycycline (100 mg twice daily) as described in that section should be started immediately and this therapy continued for 14 days. Do not wait for the characteristic rash of Rocky Mountain spotted fever or the fever pattern of Colorado tick fever to develop or for a firm diagnosis of either to be established by a physician.

Dengue

Dengue—also called Breakbone Fever or Dandy Fever—is a viral infection caused by a virus (Group B arbovirus or flavivirus) and is spread by bites from *Aedes aegypti* mosquito. Dengue is endemic throughout the tropics and subtropics. Check for latest information on active disease areas and countries receptive to this disease by contacting IAMAT for specific country update (see Appendix B).

After an incubation period of 3 to 15 (usually 5 to 8) days, there is a sudden onset of fever (104° F, 40° C), chills, headache, low back ache, pain behind the eyes with movement of the eyes, extreme aching in the legs and joints. The eyes are red and a transient flushing or pale pink rash occurs, mostly on the face. There is a relatively slow pulse rate for the temperature (see page 25). The fever lasts 48 to 96 hours, followed by 24 hours of no fever and a sense of well being. A second rapid temperature increase occurs, but generally not as high as the first. A bright rash spreads from the arms/legs to the trunk, but generally not the face. Palms and soles may be bright red and swollen. There is a severe headache and other body aches as well. The fever, rash, and headache constitute the "dengue triad." The illness lasts for weeks, but mortality is nil. Treatment is rest and the use of pain and fever medication. A condition called Dengue hemorrhagic fever shock syndrome is lethal and occurs in patients younger than 10 usually and generally infants under 1 year of age. Dengue may be confused with Colorado tick fever, typhus, yellow fever, or other hemorrhagic fevers such as the Ebola virus or Rift Valley fever in Africa.

Echinococcus

Also called *hydatid disease,* the echinococcus infection is caused by the larval stage of a tapeworm found in dogs (with sheep as an intermediate host), or in wolves in wilderness areas (with moose as the intermediate host). This disease is worldwide, but most commonly a problem in Europe, Russia, Japan, Alaska, Canada, and the continental United States, particularly Isle Royal in Lake Superior. When ingested by sheep, moose, or humans, the eggs form embryos that pass through the intestinal circulation into the liver and sometimes beyond into the lungs, brain, kidneys, and other tissue. There a fluid-filled cyst forms, which contains scolices, brood capsules, and second generation (daughter) cysts containing infectious scolices. The hydatid cysts maintain their presence, sometimes bursting and spreading in a malignant fashion causing destruction of liver, lung, and other critical tissues. After remaining without symptoms for decades, abdominal pain, jaundice, or chest pain and coughing may commence.

If the intermediate host is eaten by a carnivore (dog, wolf, or man), the infectious scolices are released into the gastrointestinal tract, where they develop into adult worms and the life cycle continues.

Most hydatid disease is from a particular tapeworm known as *Echinococcus granulosis*, but a rapidly progressive form develops when infection is caused by the *Echinococcus multilocularis* tapeworm. This tapeworm is carried primarily by foxes and domestic dogs and cats. Numerous small cysts form that multiply rapidly. The result is often fatal. There is no adequate medical treatment; attempts at surgical removal of multiple cysts are the only reliable hope for cure.

Ehrlichiosis

Since its discovery in 1987, more than 250 cases of ehrlichiosis have been reported from 21 states, principally Oklahoma, Missouri, and Georgia. The time of greatest risk is May through July. This is a rickettsial infection caused by *Ehrlichia chaffeensis* and is spread by several species of ticks.

The incubation time ranges from 1 to 21 days (mean 7 days). It presents with high fever and headache, with other common symptoms being tiredness, nausea, vomiting, muscle ache, and loss of appetite. Twenty percent of victims develop a rash, but this rash is seldom on the feet or hands. This disease can range from mild flu-like symptoms or in its extreme can be fatal.

The drug of choice is doxycycline 100 mg twice daily for 10 days.

Encephalitis

Encephalitis from Group A Arbovirus (Western equine encephalitis, Eastern equine encephalitis, Venezuelan equine encephalitis) in the United States and Canada, and from Group B Arbovirus (St. Louis encephalitis) in the United States can be prevented by liberal use of repellent and covering exposed areas with netting or clothing to prevent bites from infected mosquitos. Symptoms of these illnesses include high fever (104° F, 40° C) and generally headache, stiff neck, and vomiting and, at times, diarrhea. These cases can be fatal and require evacuation to medical help. Cool the patient with external means (cool water, fanning), and the use of aspirin or Mobigesic. The disease occurs in epidemics; be very careful with mosquito exposure when the disease becomes prevalent.

Giardiasis

Intestinal infection by *Giardia lamblia*, a single-cell parasite, *giardiasis* or *beaver fever* is becoming a significant problem in wilderness travel in the United States and is a very common cause of traveler's diarrhea. The stools of infected individuals contain the infective cyst form of the parasite. These cysts can live in water for longer than 3 months. Other mammalian vectors, such as the beaver, are responsible for much of the wilderness spread of this disease.

In the active disease, the trophozoite form attaches itself to the small bowel by means of a central sucker. Multiplication is by binary fission, or division. Approximately 2 weeks after ingestion of the cysts there is either a gradual or abrupt onset of persistent watery diarrhea, which usually resolves in 1 to 2 weeks, but may persist less severely for several months. Abdominal pain, bloating, nausea, and weight loss from malabsorption may occur. Giardiasis is often without symptoms at all and a chronic carrier state exists. In the United States about 4% of stools submitted for parasitology examination contain *G. lamblia* cysts.

Diagnosis is by finding cysts in stools or trophozoites from gastric suction or the "string test" from the duodenum. This latter test is performed by having the patient swallow a string, allowing the far end to pass into the first part of the bowel, or duodenum. When the string is pulled out, a microscopic examination may demonstrate the presence of trophozoites. In active disease the cysts are routinely secreted, but in the chronic carrier state repeated stool examinations (at least three) are required to provide a 95% accuracy of test results.

Treatment is with one of several drugs available in the United States, the most commonly used being Flagyl (metronidazol) 250 mg 3 times daily for 5 days. A better drug is quinacrine 100 mg 3 times daily for 5 days. Prevention is by proper filtration of water, adequate chemical treatment, or heating water to 150° F (66° C). See page 83 for a full discussion of water treatment.

Hantavirus

Hantavirus was the cause of death among members of the Navaho Indian Nation in New Mexico in 1993. The virus has been identified in serum samples from 42 people in 12 states with the greatest concentration in southwestern United States. It is caught by inhaling dust contaminated with feces from an infected deer mouse (*Peromyscus maniculatus*).

The onset of illness is a period of fever, muscle ache, and cough, followed by an abrupt onset of acute respiratory distress. The mortality rate has been 60%! There is no specific treatment available. Avoiding breathing dust that may contain the contaminated mouse feces is the preventative measure.

Hepatitis A

A viral infection of the liver, hepatitis A (infectious hepatitis) has wordwide distribution. It is transmitted by ingestion of infected feces, in water supplies contaminated by human sewage, food handled by persons with poor hygiene, or contaminated food such as raw shellfish grown in impure water. Contaminated milk, even infusion of infected blood products (see hepatitis B), can spread this disease.

The period from the time of exposure to the appearance of symptoms takes 15 to 50 days. The disease can range from minor flu-like symptoms to fatal liver disease. Most cases resolve favorably within 6 to 12 weeks. Symptoms start abruptly with fever, lethargy, and nausea. Occasionally a rash develops. A characteristic loss of taste for cigarettes is frequent. In 3 to 10 days the urine turns dark, followed by jaundice, with yellowing of the whites of the eyes and the skin. The stool may turn light colored. There is frequently itching and joint pain. The jaundice peaks within one to two weeks and fades during the two-to-four week recovery phase. The hepatitis A patient stops shedding virus in the stool prior to the jaundice developing, and is therefore not contagious by the time the diagnosis is normally made. Personal hygiene helps prevent spreading, but isolation of the patient is not strictly required.

In most cases no specific treatment is required. After a few days to 2 weeks appetite generally returns and bed confinement is no longer required, even though jaundice still remains. The best guideline is the disappearance of the lethargy and feeling of illness that appeared in the first stages of the disease. Restrictions of diet have no value, but a low fat diet is generally more palatable.

If profound prostration occurs, the trip should be terminated for the patient and he should be placed under medical care. If possible, unimmunized contacts should receive gamma-globulin 0.02 ml/kg IM. Anyone traveling outside of North America, Northern Europe, Australia, and New Zealand should be immunized with hepatitis A vaccine (see *immunization,* Appendix B).

Hepatitis B

Another viral infection of the liver, Hepatitis B (serum hepatitis) is also worldwide in distribution. Transmission is primarily through infusion of infected blood products, sexual contact, use of contaminated needles, syringes, or even sharing contaminated razor blades. Dental procedures, acupuncture, and ear piercing and tattooing with contaminated equipment will also spread this disease.

Incubation period from time of exposure to the development of symptoms is longer than with hepatitis A, namely 30 to 180 days. The symptoms are similar, but the onset is less abrupt and the incidence of fever is lower. There is a greater chance of developing chronic hepatitis (5 to 10% of cases). Mortality is higher, especially in elderly patients where it ranges from 10 to 15%.

Immunization is available and is very effective (see Appendix B). This immunization is usually recommended for persons engaging in foreign travel and certainly should be obtained by anyone working in a medical or dental capacity anywhere in the world.

Hepatitis C

A form of hepatitis, with similar manifestations to hepatitis B, has been designated as hepatitis C (formerly "Non-A, Non-B" since blood tests for evidence of exposure to those virus particles was not previously found). The transmission is probably the same as for hepatitis B. Incubation period is from less than 2 weeks, to more than 25 weeks, with an average of 7 weeks for the development of clinical disease. There is immunization available and no specific treatment.

Hepatitis D

Hepatitis D, or the "delta agent," can only infect a person who has hepatitis B. The presence of this mutated RNA particle causes the infection to be more fulminant. It spreads only by contaminated needle use.

Hepatitis E

An epidemic form of hepatitis (that is not A or C) has been termed hepatitis E. Spread by ingestion of contaminated food or water, the incubation period from time of contact ranges from 2 to 9 weeks, with a mean of 45 days. The disease mimics hepatitis A. The fatality rate in pregnant women is highest, about 20%. Outbreaks have been confirmed throughout developing areas of the old world. There is no immunization available.

Hepatitis G

A new virus has been identified as the hepatitis G virus. A member of the family *Flaviviridae,* it can be spread by blood borne and sexual transmission, just as with hepatitis B. There is no immunization available.

Lyme Disease

Lyme disease is caused by a spirochete, *Borrelia burgdorferi.* The disease lives in various mammals, but is transmitted to humans by the bite of several species of ticks. The disease is most common in the Northeast, extending through Connecticut and Massachusetts down to Maryland; in Wisconsin and Minnesota; throughout the states of California and Oregon; in various south Atlantic and south central states; with cases reported from 43 of the lower 48 states. A map showing the reported incidence of Lyme disease per county by state within the United States is located on my Web site. It has been found in other countries as well, from the former Soviet Union, China, Australia, and Japan to several European countries.

The disease goes through several phases. In stage one, after an incubation of 3 days to a month, probably 95% of victims develop a circular lesion in the area of the bite. It has a clear to pink center, raised border, is painless, and ranges from 1 to 23 inches in diameter. There are usually several such patches. The patient feels lethargic, has headache, muscle and joint pain, and enlarged lymph nodes. In stage two 10% to 15% of patients can develop a meningitis, less than 10% develop heart problems. Symptoms may last for months, but are generally self-limited. Approximately 60% enter stage three, the development of actual arthritis. Frequently a knee is involved. The swelling can be impressive. Stage three can start abruptly several weeks to 2 years after the onset of the initial rash.

Treatment of stage one Lyme disease is tetracycline, such as doxycycline 100 mg taken twice daily for 20 days. Alternate drugs are penicillin and erythromycin. Treatment of choice for stages two and three Lyme disease consists of Rocephin 2 gram given IV daily for 14 to 21 days.

One manifestation of Lyme disease is the development of a facial paralysis on one side, called Bell's palsy. The involved side is expressionless since the patient is unable to move the muscles of the forehead, around the eye, and so on. While there are other causes of Bell's palsy, in North America this problem must be considered as Lyme disease until ruled out by a physician. Treatment of Bell's palsy caused by Lyme disease is with oral antibiotic for 21 days.

Malaria

Human malaria is caused by four species of a protozoa: *Plasmodium falciparum, P. vivax, P. Ovale,* and *P. malariae.* The infection is acquired from the bite of an infected female Anopheles mosquito. It may also be spread by blood transfusion. Falciparum malaria is the most serious. While all forms of this disease make people ill and may be lethal, *P. falciparum* is the one that kills.

Regions of the world where malaria may be acquired are subSaharan Africa, parts of Mexico and Central America, Haiti, parts of South America, the Middle East, the Indian subcontinent, and Southeast Asia. Resistance to chloroquine by the deadly *P. falciparum* has become widespread. For travelers in resistant areas the current prophylactic medication is Larium (mefloquine) 250 mg 1 tablet weekly, starting 1 week prior to departure and continuing for 4 weeks after return. Persons traveling to remote malarious areas should also consider taking 3 tablets of the drug Fansidar (pyrimethamine-sulfadoxine) once as a presumptive treatment in case the symptoms of malaria develop (ache, fever, or any questionable flu-like symptoms). Also seek medical help as soon as possible. Persons with a sulfa allergy cannot take this drug. An alternate drug regimen, especially necessary when *P. falciparum* becomes resistant to mefloquine, is the use of doxycycline 100 mg to be taken once daily for prevention.

In areas with relapsing malaria (*P. vivax* and *P. ovale*), primaquine should be taken 1 tablet daily during the last 2 weeks of chloroquine therapy. This is usually appropriate for anyone faced with long exposure in areas with a high concentration of these strains of malaria. IAMAT (see Appendix B) provides the percentage of *P. falciparum* versus *P. vivax* and *P. ovale* as well as current information on resistance to chloroquine for each country.

Meningococcal Meningitis

This acute bacterial infection caused by *Neisseria meningitidis* results in inflammation the brain and central nervous system. Many cases are without symptoms or consist of a mild upper respiratory illness. Severe cases begin with sudden fever, sore throat, chills, headache, stiff neck, nausea, and vomiting. Within 24 to 48 hours the victim becomes drowsy, mentally confused, followed by convulsions, coma, and death. Immediate and appropriately large doses of the proper antibiotic are critical to save the patient's life (the Wilderness Medical Kit only has Rocephin, which must be given in large amounts: one gram IM twice daily). The disease is spread by contact with the nasal secretions of infected persons (sneezing and coughing).

While the disease is found worldwide, large epidemics are more common in tropical countries, especially sub-Saharan Africa in the dry season, New Delhi (India), and Nepal.

In 80% of healthy young adults bacterial meningitis is caused by the meningococci bacteria discussed in this section or by a pneumococci bacterium. Vaccines are available against both of these organisms (see Appendix B).

Plague

Plague is caused by a bacterium (*Yersinia pestis*) that infects wild rodents in many parts of the world, including the western United States and parts of South America, Africa, and Asia. Epidemics occur when domestic rats become infected and spread the disease to man. Bubonic plague is transmitted by infected fleas, while pneumonic plague is spread directly to other people by coughing. Plague is accompanied by fever, enlarged lymph nodes (bubonic plague), and less commonly pneumonia (pneumonic plague). Treatment is with doxycycline 100 mg twice daily. Treat fever as necessary. Isolate patient, particularly if coughing. Drainage of abscesses (buboes) may be necessary (see page 115). Exposed persons should be watched for 10 days, but incubation is usually 2 to 6 days. Only travelers planning long stays in areas where a local epidemic is raging are at enough risk to consider using plague vaccine (see Appendix B).

Rabies

Rabies can be transmitted on the North American continent by several species of mammals, namely skunk, bat, fox, coyote, raccoon, bobcat, and wolf. Obviously, if removing an animal from a trap, jogging past an animal, separating mother from child, or taking food from a critter causes an attack, the most likely cause is not rabies. An attack by a wounded animal is cause for concern, as the animal may be wounded due to loss of coordination from rabies. Any unprovoked attack by one of these mammals should be considered an attack by a rabid animal. Dogs and cats in the United States have a low incidence of rabies. Information from local departments of health will indicate if rabies is currently of concern in your area. Animals whose bites have never caused rabies in humans in the United States are livestock (cattle, sheep, horse), rabbits, gerbils, chipmunks, squirrels, rats, and mice. A significant epidemic of raccoon rabies has now extended from Florida to Connecticut, with isolated reports from New Hampshire and Ohio showing an expansion of this epidemic north and west. Hawaii is the only rabies free state.

In the United States there have been 36 human deaths from rabies reported since 1980, 12 of which were acquired during foreign travel. In India 40,000 to 50,000 people die yearly from rabies, with a large incidence in the other developing countries of Asia, Africa, and Latin America.

In many foreign countries the bite of a cat or dog should be considered rabid. Countries free of rabies are England, Australia, Japan, and parts of the Caribbean. In Europe the red fox and bats are the animals most often rabid, with documented cases spreading to dogs, cats, cattle, and deer. Canada's rabies occurs mostly in foxes and skunks in the province of Ontario. Mongoose rabies is found in South Africa and the Caribbean islands of Cuba, Puerto Rico, Hispaniola, and Grenada.

The treatment for rabies is rabies immune globulin 20 IU/kg, with half infiltrated around the wound and the remaining half in the gluteal area (upper outer quadrant of the bottom) and human diploid cell vaccine (HDCV) 1 ml given IM in the shoulder on days 0, 3, 7, 14, and 28.

The incubation period in a human is 1 to 2 months. Rabies is a vicious, usually fatal disease once it develops clinically. Because of this, there is generous use of rabies vaccine and immune globulin. Approximately 16,000 to 39,000 people are vaccinated in the United States yearly to prevent this disease. Persons having to work with potentially rabid animal populations can be immunized with the vaccine and given yearly booster shots. It is possible to obtain the disease by merely being contaminated with the saliva or blood of an infected animal if it comes in contact with a break in the skin or mucous membranes, and possibly even by breathing in dust infected with the virus. Two cases of human rabies have been attributed to airborne exposures in a bat cave in Texas. Note that 58% of human rabies cases in the United States have been from bats.

Relapsing Fever

This bacterial infection is caused by several species of *Borrelia spirochete* and is spread by body lice in Asia, Africa, and Europe, or by soft body ticks in the Americas (including the western United States), Asia, Africa, and Europe.

Symptoms occur 3 to 11 days from contact with the tick or louse vector and start with an abrupt onset of chills, headache, muscular pains, and sometimes vomiting. A rash may appear and small hemorrhages present under the skin surface. The fever remains high from 3 to 5 days, then clears suddenly. After 1 to 2 weeks a somewhat milder relapse begins. Jaundice is more common during relapse. The illness again clears, but 2 to 10 similar episodes reoccur at intervals of 1 to 2 weeks until immunity fully develops.

Antibiotics are available for effective treatment. Mortality is low, less than 5% in healthy adults. Treatment is with doxycycline 100 mg twice daily for 5 to 10 days. Personal hygiene is effective in preventing louse-borne disease, while control of ticks with insect repellent and frequent body checks and tick removal minimize the chance of tick-borne disease. Unlike many tick-borne diseases that will not spread to humans unless the tick as been attached for longer than two days, relapsing fever can be caught soon after attachment.

Rocky Mountain Spotted Fever

This is an acute and serious infection caused by a microorganism called *Rickettsia rickettsii* and transmitted by Ixodid (hard-shelled) ticks. It is most common in the states of North Carolina, Virginia, Maryland, the Rocky Mountain States, and the state of Washington. The peak incidence of cases is from May to September. Onset of infection is abrupt, after a 3 to 12-day incubation period (average 7 days from the tick bite). Fever reaches 103° to 104° F (40° C) within 2 days. There is considerable headache, chills, and muscle pain at the onset. In 4 days a rash appears on wrists, ankles, soles, palms, and then spreads to the trunk. Initially pink, this rash turns to dark blotches and even ulcers in severe cases. Any suspected case of Rocky Mountain spotted fever should be considered a medical emergency. Do not wait for the rash to develop;

rather start the patient on antibiotics from the Rx kit. Give doxycycline 100 mg, 1 tablet every 12 hours and keep on this dosage schedule for 14 days. This is a drug of choice and its early use can cut the death rate from 20% to nearly zero. Prevention is by the careful removal of ticks, the use of insect repellent and protective clothing.

Schistosomiasis

Blood trematodes or flukes are responsible for schistosomiasis (*Bilharziasis, Safari Fever*). The eggs are deposited in fresh water and hatch into motile miracidia, which infect snails. After developing in the snails, active cercariae emerge, which can penetrate exposed human skin. Swimming, wading, or drinking fresh water must be avoided in infected areas.

Schistosoma mansoni is found in tropical Africa, part of Venezuela, several Caribbean islands, the Guianas, Brazil, and the Middle East. *S. japonicum* is encountered in China, Japan, the Philippines, and Southeast Asia. *S. haematobium* is in Africa, the Middle East, and small portions of India and islands in the Indian Ocean. The former two species are excreted in the stools and the latter in urine. Shedding may occur for years. No isolation is required of patients. Specific treatments for the various species are available. Check for latest information on dangerous areas by contacting IAMAT (see Appendix B).

Initial penetration of the skin causes an itchy rash. After entry, the organism enters the bloodstream, migrates through the lungs, and eventually lodges in the blood vessels draining either the gut or the bladder, depending upon the species. While the worms are maturing the victim will have fever, lethargy, cough, rash, abdominal pain, and often nausea. In acute infections caused by *S. mansoni* and *S. japonicum*, victims develop a mucoid, bloody diarrhea and tender liver enlargement. Chronic infection leads to fibrosis of the liver with distention of the abdomen. In *S. haematobium* infections the bladder becomes inflamed and eventually fibrotic. Symptoms include painful urination, urgency, blood in urine, and pelvic pain.

Tapeworms

Three species of tapeworms infect humans: *Taenia saginata* larvae found in beef, *Taenia solium* in pork, and *Diphyllobothrium latum* in fish. In all three the human ingests undercooked flesh of the host animal acquiring the infective cysts.

The beef tapeworm can be huge, forming lengths of 10 to 30 feet inside the human host. It is common in Mexico, South America, Eastern Europe, the Middle East, and Africa. Symptoms can include stomach pain, weight loss, and diarrhea, but frequently the human host has no clue of the infestation.

The pork tapeworm infects its victims in South America, Eastern Europe, Russia, and Asia. Generally it is without symptoms; at times vague abdominal complaints are noted. A complication of this disease is cystocercosis: The tapeworm larvae penetrate the human intestinal wall—after the human drinks infected water—and invade body tissues, frequently skeletal muscle and the brain. There they mature into cystic masses. After several years the cysts degenerate and produce local inflammatory reactions that can then cause convulsions, visual problems, or mental disturbances. In this case the human replaces the pig in the maturation cycle of the tapeworm and it is the human flesh that is contaminated by the tapeworm cyst. This is an unlucky break for the involved human and any cannibals whom he might meet. Any water filtration or purification system can prevent cystocercosis.

Fish tapeworm occurs worldwide, but is particularly a hazard in Scandinavia and the Far East. A single tapeworm, usually without symptoms, develops. The worm's absorption of vitamin B-12 may cause pernicious anemia in the host.

Tetanus

Caused by a bacterium, *Clostridium tetani*, that is located worldwide, most cases of tetanus occur from very minor wounds, such as a papercut, rather than rusty barbed wire as so many people think. In fact, a hiker on the Appalachian Trail got tetanus from a blister on his heel and inadequate immunization. Onset is gradual, with an incubation period of 2 to 50 (usually 5 to 10) days. The earliest symptom is stiffness of the jaw, then sore throat, stiff muscles, headache, low-grade fever, and muscle spasm. As the disease progresses, the patient is unable to open her jaw and the facial muscles may be fixed in a smile with elevated eyebrows. Painful generalized spasms of muscles occur with minor disturbances such as drafts, noise, or someone jarring the patient's bed. Death from loss of respiratory muscle function, or even unknown causes, may ensue. The disease is frequently fatal.

Prevention is obtained by adequate immunization (see Appendix B).

Tick Paralysis

Five species of tick in North America produce a neurotoxin in their saliva that can paralyze their victims. Most cases are found in the Pacific Northwest, Rocky Mountain states, and 7 southern states, as well as Australia. Spring and summer are the times of highest risk.

The toxin is usually carried by an engorged, pregnant tick. Symptoms begin 2 to 7 days after the tick begins feeding. Throughout the ordeal the patient's mental function is usually spared. Symptoms start as weakness in the legs, which progressively ascends until the entire body is paralyzed over several hours to days. At times the condition presents as ataxia (loss of coordination) without muscle weakness.

The diagnosis is made by finding an embedded tick. After removing the tick, symptoms resolve in hours to days, rarely longer. Untreated tick paralysis can be fatal with mortality rates of 10 to 12%.

Trichinosis

Trichinosis is caused by eating improperly cooked meat infected with the cysts of this parasite. It is most common in pigs, bears (particularly polar bears), and some marine mammals. Nausea and diarrhea or intestinal cramping may appear within 1 to 2 days, but it generally takes 7 days after indigestion. Swelling of the eyelids is very characteristic on the 11th day. Afterwards, muscle soreness, fever, pain in the eyes, and subconjunctival hemorrhage (see page 45) develop. If enough contaminated food is ingested this can be a fatal disease. Most symptoms disappear in 3 months.

Treatment is with pain medication (Percogesic from the Non-Rx Oral Medication Module or Lorcet 10/650 from the Rx Oral Medication Module). The use of steroids such as Decadron (20 mg/day for 3 or 4 days, followed by reduced dosage over the next 10 days) is indicated in severe cases. Thiabendazole is a specific drug for use in this condition, given orally in doses of 25 mg/kg of body weight twice daily for 5 to 10 days. The best prevention is cooking suspected meat at 150° F (66° C) for 30 minutes for each pound of meat.

African Sleeping Sickness

Two species of trypanosomes cause African sleeping sickness (African Trypanosomiasis), which is transmitted by the bite of the tsetse fly. The severity of the disease depends upon the species encountered. The infection is confined to the area of Africa between 15 degrees north and 20 degrees south of the equator—the exact distribution of the tsetse fly. Humans are the only reservoir of *Trypanosoma gambiense* found in West and Central Africa, while wild game is the principal reservoir of *T. rhodesiense* of East Africa.

T. gambiense infection starts with a nodule or a chancre that appears briefly at the site of a tsetse fly bite. Generalized illness appears months to years later and is characterized by lymph node enlargement at the back of the neck and intermittent fever. Months to years after this development, invasion of the central nervous system may occur, noted by behavioral changes, headache, loss of appetite, backache, hallucinations, delusions, and sleeping. In *T. rhodesiense* infection the generalized illness begins 5 to 14 days after the nodule or chancre develops. It is much more intense than the Gambian variety and may include acute central nervous system and cardiac symptoms, fever, and rapid weight loss. It has a high rate of mortality. If untreated, death usually occurs within 1 year. Specific, but frequently toxic, therapy is available.

Chagas' Disease

Chagas' disease (American Trypanosomiasis) caused by *Trypanosoma cruzi*, a protozoan hemoflagellate, is transmitted through the feces of a brown insect called the "kissing bug" or "assassin bug" in North America. This bug is a member of the family *Reduviidae*. A name popular in South America is "vinchuca," derived from a word which means "one who lets himself fall down." These bugs live in palm trees or thatching in native huts, and like to drop on their victims while sleeping, on the face or exposed arms. When biting victims, the bug defecates. The itch of the wound causes bitten patients to scratch the wound, rubbing the feces into the bite site, thus causing the inoculation of the infectious agent.

This disease is located in parts of South and Central America. Check for latest information on dangerous areas by contacting IAMAT (see Appendix B). At first this disease may have no symptoms. A "chagoma" or red nodule develops at the site of the original infection. This area may then lose its pigmentation. After 1 to 2 weeks, a firm swelling of one eyelid occurs, known as Romana's sign. The swelling becomes purplish in color, and lymph node swelling in front of the ear on the same side may occur. In a few days a fever develops, with generalized lymph node swelling. Rapid heartrate, spleen and liver enlargement, swelling of the legs, and meningitis or encephalitis may occur. Serious conditions also can include acute heart failure. In most cases, however, the illness subsides in about 3 months and the patient appears to live a normal life. The disease continues, however, slowly destroying the heart until 10 to 20 years later chronic congestive heart failure becomes apparent. The underlying cause may never be known, especially in a traveler who has left the endemic area. In some areas of Brazil, the disease attacks the colon, causing flaccid enlargement with profound constipation. This disease is a leading cause of death in South America, generally due to heart failure. As many as 15 million people in South America may be infected. Special blood tests are available through state Boards of Health and Centers for Disease Control and Prevention. Supportive treatment is given during acute disease and specific treatments are being developed.

Tuberculosis

Tuberculosis is caused by one of two bacteria, *Mycobacterium tuberculosis* or *M. bovis*. The infection results in a very chronic illness that can reactivate many years after it has been apparently killed. In the United States there are 20,000 new cases, with 1,800 deaths yearly. Worldwide there are 8 to 10 million new cases, with 2 to 3 million deaths yearly. This disease is spread primarily by inhalation of infected droplets. The disease also spreads by drinking infected milk or eating infected dairy products such as butter.

Active disease usually develops within a year of contact. The early symptoms of fever, night sweats, lethargy, and weight loss can be so gradual that they are initially ignored. Tuberculosis usually infects the lungs, but it can spread throughout the body causing neurological damage, bone infections, and overwhelming infection. Diagnosis is usually made with a chest x-ray.

A traveler heading into an area with epidemic tuberculosis should have a pre- and post-trip TB skin test. A negative TB skin test does not exclude a diagnosis of TB, but it can be a very useful aid in evaluating the chance that a traveler has contacted tuberculosis. A TB test should be repeated about 6 months after returning from the trip to provide adequate chance for it to react. Specific antibiotic therapy is available. Immunization is available, but not usually used in the United States (see Appendix B).

Tularemia

Tularemia (Rabbit Fever, Deer Fly Fever) can be contracted through exposure to ticks, deer flies, or mosquitos. Cuts can be infected when working with rabbit pelts. Eating improperly cooked infected rabbits can result in onset. Similarly, muskrats, foxes, squirrels, mice, and rats can spread the disease via direct contact with their carcasses. Stream water may become contaminated by these animals.

An ulcer appears when a wound is involved and lymph nodes become enlarged first in nearby areas and then throughout the body. Pneumonia normally develops. The disease lasts 4 weeks in untreated cases. Mortality in treated cases is almost zero, while in untreated cases it ranges from 6 to 30%.

Treatment of choice is streptomycin, but the doxycycline suggested for the Rx Oral/Topical Medication Module works extremely well. The average adult would require an initial dose of 2 tablets, followed by 1 tablet every 12 hours. Continue therapy for 5 to 7 days after the fever has been broken.

Typhoid Fever

Caused by the bacterium *Salmonella typhi,* typhoid fever is spread by contaminated food and dairy products. Prevention is proper food storage, the thorough cooking of food, and avoidance of unrefrigerated dairy products.

The disease is characterized by headache, chills, loss of appetite, backache, constipation, nosebleed, and tenderness of the abdomen to palpation. The temperature rises daily for 7 to 10 days. The fever is maintained at a high level for 7 to 19 more days, then drops over the next 10 days. With typhoid fever, a pulse rate of only 84 may occur with a temperature of 104° F (40° C), when one might otherwise expect a pulse rate of over 120. Between the 7th and 10th days of the illness, rose-colored splotches, which blanche when pressure is applied, appear in 10% of patients.

The drug of choice for treating this illness is Rocephin, given 30 mg/kg of body weight/day IM in 2 divided doses per day for 2 weeks. An oral drug that can be used is Levaquin 500 mg given once daily. Diarrhea may be severe in the latter stages of this illness. Replacement of fluids is especially important during the phases of high fever or diarrhea (see page 82). Patients with relapses should be given another five day course of the antibiotic. Immunization prior to departure to endemic areas is useful in preventing or curtailing the severity of this infection (see page 236).

Endemic Typhus, Flea Borne

This disease is also known as murine typhus, rat-flea typhus, New World typhus, Malaya typhus, and urban typhus. It is one of several diseases caused by *rickettsia,* which resemble both viral and bacterial infections. Other diseases caused by this order are Rocky Mountain spotted fever, Q-fever, trench fever, and the various typhus diseases. Endemic typhus is due to *Rickettsia typhi.* It is located worldwide, including the southern Atlantic and Gulf Coast states of the United States. It is spread to humans through infected rat flea feces.

After an incubation period of 6 to 18 days (mean 10), shaking chills, fever, and headache develop. A rash forms primarily on the trunk, but fades fairly rapidly. The fever lasts about 12 days. This is a mild disease and fatalities are rare. Antibiotic treatment with doxycycline 100 mg given twice daily is very effective. Prevention is directed toward vector (rat and flea) control.

Epidemic Typhus, Louse-Borne

This malady is also called classic typhus, European typhus, and jail fever. It killed 3 million people during World War II. On the positive side, no American traveler has contracted this disease since 1950. It is most likely to be encountered in mountainous regions of Mexico, Central and South America, the Balkans, eastern Europe, Africa, and many countries of Asia. The causative agent is *Rickettsia prowazekii*, which is transmitted by infected lice.

Following a 7 to 14 day incubation period, there is a sudden onset of high fever (104° F, 40° C), which remains at a high level, with a usual morning decrease, for about 2 weeks. There is an intense headache. A light pink rash appears on the 4th to 6th day, soon becoming dark red. There is low blood pressure, pneumonia, mental confusion, and bruising in severe cases. Mortality is rare in children less than 10 years of age, but may reach greater than 60% in those over 50. Antibiotics, such as doxycycline 100 mg twice daily, are very effective if given early in the disease. Prevention is proper hygiene and delousing when needed. A vaccine was formerly made in the United States, but is no longer available and is not needed due to the low incidence observed in American travelers.

Yellow Fever

An arbovirus, yellow fever is found in tropical areas of South and Central America and Africa. This viral disease is contracted by the bite of the *Aedes aegypti* mosquito (and other species). Onset, about 2 weeks after the bite, is sudden, with a fever of 102° to 104° F (40° C). The pulse is usually rapid the first day, but becomes slow by the second day. In mild cases the fever falls suddenly 2 to 5 days after onset. This remission lasts for hours to several days. Next the fever returns, but the pulse remains slow. Jaundice, vomiting of black blood, and severe loss of protein in the urine (causing it to become foamy) occurs during this stage. Hemorrhages may be noted in the mouth and skin (petechiae). The patient is confused and senses are dulled. Delirium, convulsions, and coma occur before death in approximately 10% of cases. If the patient is to survive, this last febrile episode lasts from 3 to 9 days. With remission the patient is well, with no after-effects from the disease.

Immunization is available and required or recommended for travel to many countries (see Appendix B).

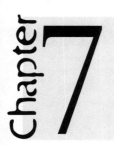

Chapter

7 Environmental Injuries

While ankle sprains, blisters, and diarrhea are the most common problems facing the wilderness traveler, environmental conditions pose the most likely threat to life★ (other than the highway system used to reach the trailhead). Foremost among these dangers is hypothermia. Death from heat exposure is still the second leading cause of death among high school athletes (discounting the highway). Unless you live

★Couse, J.C., Josephs D. "Health Care of Appalachian Trail Hikers." *Journal of Family Medicine* 1993; 36:521–525.

right on the Pacific Coast, lightning can do more than scare you. And for the many of us trekking vertically, high altitude illnesses are potentially miserable, even lethal, experiences.

Hypothermia

The term *hypothermia* refers to the lowering of the body's core temperature to 95° F (35° C); *profound hypothermia* is a core temperature lower than 90° F (32° C). Another important point is that in the wilderness setting, the term hypothermia applies to two distinctly different diseases. *Chronic hypothermia* is the slow onset of hypothermia in the outdoors traveler exposed to conditions too cold to be protected by his equipment; *acute,* or *immersion, hypothermia* is the rapid onset of hypothermia of a person immersed in cold water.

In acute hypothermia—when the onset of cold core temperature takes less than two hours—the body cannot produce the complex physiological responses that it is capable of if it had more time. In chronic hypothermia—when body temperature takes 6 hours or longer to arrive at the cold core—the responses are quite dramatic and include profound dehydration, exhaustion, and complex chemical changes in the blood. The ideal treatment is quite different in the hospital setting, but in the field our treatment options are reduced to basic techniques of preventing further heat loss and some passive reheating maneuvers.*

Chronic Hypothermia

You do not have to be in a bitterly cold setting to die of hypothermia. In fact most chronic hypothermia deaths occur in the 30° F (0° C) to 50° F (10° C) range. This temperature range places almost all of North America in a high risk-status all year long. To survive hypothermia: be prepared to prevent it, recognize it if it occurs, and know how to treat it. Dampness and wind are the most devastating factors to be considered: dampness can reduce the insulation of clothing and cause evaporative heat loss, and the increased convection heat loss caused by wind can readily strip away body energy, the so-called "wind chill" effect.

Factors important in preventing hypothermia are a high level of pretrip physical conditioning, adequate nutritional and hydration status,

*Refer to Forgey, *Basic Essentials: Hypothermia,* The Globe Pequot Press, 1999, for a full discussion of the physiological changes of rapid-onset and delayed-onset hypothermia, including prevention, diagnosis, and treatment.

avoiding exhaustion, and availability of adequate insulation. There is increased risk of hypothermia in case of injury, especially shock, or if the above preventative conditions are inadequate.

An initial response to cold is *vasoconstriction,* or the clamping down of surface blood vessels. This prevents heat from being conducted to the surface by the blood and effectively increases the thicknesss of the mantle, or outer layer depth, for increased insulation. Those who become profoundly hypothermic, with a core temperature below 90° F, have concentrated their blood volume into a small inner core. The amount of dehydration in these persons can be profound, approaching 5.5 liters in someone below 90° F, equivalent to the entire circulatory volume. This fluid loss comes not only from the vascular space but also from fluid between the cells and within the cells as the body slowly adjusts to the continuing heat loss by shrinking blood circulation into the core and increasing the thickness of the mantle layer. At this point, rapid, sudden rewarming can lead to *rewarming shock.* Hospital methods of rewarming must be coupled with tight metabolic control by adjusting blood factors such as clotting, electrolytes, blood sugar levels, etc.

In chronic hypothermia rewarming shock and loss of metabolic control are the causes of death, not the so-called *after-drop phenomenon.* After-drop, or the further lowering of core temperature after rewarming has started, is due to the combination of conduction equilibration of heat and a circulation component. By far the most important aspect is conduction equilibration. This physical property of conduction results in an equilibration of thermal mass as the higher warmth of the core leaches into the colder mantle layer. The amount of after-drop that occurs is primarily dependent upon the rate of cooling prior to the rewarming process, not the method of rewarming!

The treatment of the chronic hypothermic victim is to prevent further loss of heat; this generally means providing shelter and/or more adequate clothing. The victim is exhausted and thus requires rest and food. She is dehydrated and requires fluids. If she can stand, a roaring fire can provide adequate, controlled heat. Since chronic hypothermia victims are exhausted they will not be able to exercise themselves to warmth. Exercise is a method of generating heat, as is shivering, but when energy stores are consumed, exhaustion commences and significant hypothermia will begin unless further heat loss is stopped.

Deepening hypothermia will lead to a semi-comatose state and worse. This victim needs to be evacuated and hospitalized. Wrap to prevent further heat loss and transport. Chemical heat packs, etc. can be added to the wrap to help offset further heat loss, but care must be taken not to burn the victim. If evacuation is not feasible, add heat slowly to avoid rewarming shock. Huddling the victim between two rescuers in an adequate sleeping bag may be the only alternative. On all of my expeditions into northern Canada in the winter, we always carry a set of semi-rectangular bags that can twin so that such treatment is feasible.

Acute Hypothermia

After-drop is, however, a real problem for the acute or immersion hypothermic who has had a significant exposure to cold water. As a rule of thumb, a person who has been in water of 50° F (10° C) or less for a period of 20 minutes or longer is suffering from a severe amount of heat loss. That individual's thermal mass has been so reduced that he is in potentially serious condition. He should not be allowed to move around as this will increase the blood flow to his very cold skin and facilitate a profound circulatory-induced after-drop—one that is so great as to be potentially lethal. If this same person is simply wrapped in a litter and not provided with outside heat, there is a real danger his core temperature will cool down to a lethal level because of this profound amount of heat loss.

The ideal treatment is rapid rewarming of the acute hypothermic by placing him in hot water (110° F/43° C) to allow rapid replacement of heat. The acute hypothermic may have an almost normal core temperature initially, but it is destined to drop dramatically as his body equilibrates his heat store from his core to his very cold mantle. A roaring fire can be a lifesaver. If not available, huddling two rescuers with the victim in a large sleeping bag may be the only answer—the same therapy that might have to be employed in the field treatment of chronic hypothermia under some conditions.

The person who has been immersed for less than 20 minutes in cold water can do anything he wants to rewarm. He can run around like crazy, stand by a fire, or just wrap up in warm, dry insulation. The total body thermal mass is still high enough that the temperature equilibration by both the conductive and circulatory components will not reduce the core temperature to a dangerous level.

To review, the person who has been in cold water longer than 20 minutes has experienced such a profound heat loss that allowing him to run around or even wrapping him without additional significant heat will cause a tremendous drop in his core temperature—into a lethal range. The person who is fished out of the cold water after two hours or longer must be considered as approaching chronic hypothermia. He has survived long enough that his physiological protective mechanisms have resulted in dehydration and other changes that are so complex that rapid rewarming can result in shock and death unless he is carefully monitored in a hospital setting.

Cold Water Submersion

Cold water submersion★ is always associated with asphyxiation and simultaneous hypothermia.

Asphyxiation results in brain death so that prompt rescue and immediate implementation of CPR (cardiopulmonary resuscitation) play an important role in the survival of the victim. Total submersion in cold water causes a rapid core cooling, which results in a lower oxygen demand by the brain and other body tissues and increases the chance of survival over that of a victim of warm water submersion. Full recovery after 10 to 40 minutes of submersion can occur. CPR must be continued until the body has been warmed to at least 86° F (30° C). If still unresponsive at that temperature, the victim may be considered dead. It may take several hours of CPR while the patient is being properly rewarmed to make this determination.

The rewarming process for immersion victims should not be attempted in the field. Hospital management of victims of cold water submersion is very complex. They are best transferred to centers experienced with this problem, but they will never have a chance if rescuers do not implement CPR immediately.

Cold-Stress Injuries

Frost nip

Frost nip, or very light frostbite, can be readily treated in the field if recognized early enough. This term is usually reserved for a form of superficial frostbite, but I am convinced that there really is a separate entity that should be considered *frost nip:* The skin turns pure white in a small patch, generally the tip of the nose or ear edges. When detected, cup your hands and blow on the affected parts to effect total rewarming.

★Note that there is a distinct difference between immersion and submersion: *Submersion* indicates that the victim is entirely under water; *immersion* means that the head is above water.

Under identical exposure conditions, some people are more prone to this than others. On one of my trips into subarctic Canada, a companion almost constantly frost-nipped his nose at rather mild temperatures (20° F, -7° C). We frequently had to warn him, as he seemed oblivious to the fact that the tip of his nose would repeatedly frost.

Frostbite

Frostbite is the freezing of skin tissue. The temperature of the skin must be 24° F (-4° C) before it will freeze. Risk for frostbite increases if the victim is hypothermic, dehydrated, injured, wearing tight-fitting clothing or boots, or is not removing boots and changing socks or checking his feet at least nightly.

Traditionally, several degrees of frostbite are recognized, but the treatment for all is the same. The actual degree of severity will not be known until after the patient has been treated. In the wilderness, most cases of frostbite are not identified until the area has already thawed and the blue, discolored skin is found when finally changing socks or actually looking at the area in question.

When superficial frostbite is suspected, thaw immediately so that it does not become a more serious, deep frostbite. Warm the hands by withdrawing them into the parka through the sleeves—avoid opening the front of the parka to minimize heat loss. Feet should be thawed against a companion or cupped in your hands in a roomy sleeping bag or other insulated environment.

The specific therapy for a deeply frozen extremity is rapid thawing in warm water (approximately 110° F, 43° C). This thawing may take 20–30 minutes, but it should be continued until all paleness of the tops of the fingers or toes has turned to pink or burgundy red, but no longer. This will be very painful and will require pain medication (Rx Lorcet 10/650 1 tablet, nasal Stadol, or injectable Nubain will probably be required).

Avoid opening the blisters that form. Do not cut skin away, but allow the digits to auto-amputate over the next 3 months. Blisters will usually last 2 to 3 weeks and must be treated with care to prevent infections (best done in a hospital with gloved attendants).

A black carapace will form in *severe frostbite*. This is actually a form of dry gangrene. The carapace will gradually fall off with amazingly good healing beneath. Efforts to hasten the carapace removal generally result in infection, delay in healing, and increased tissue loss. *Leave these black-*

ened areas alone. The black carapace separation can take over 6 months, but it is worth the wait. Without surgical interference, most frostbite wounds heal in 6 months to a year. All persons heading into the bush should already have had their tetanus booster (within the previous 10 years). Treat for shock with elevation of feet and lowering of the head, as shock will frequently occur when these people enter a warm environment.

Once the victim has been thawed, very careful management of the thawed part is required. Refreezing will result in substantial tissue loss and this must be avoided. The patient sometimes becomes a stretcher case if the foot is involved, but not always. For that reason, it may be necessary to leave the foot or leg(s) frozen and allow the victim to walk back to the evacuation point or facility where the thawing will take place, realizing that the amount of damage is increasing the longer the area remains frozen. Early, rapid thawing is essential to minimize tissue loss. Do not allow the extremity to remain frozen unless it is essential to preserve life. Peter Freuchen, the great Greenland explorer, once walked days and miles keeping one leg frozen, knowing that when the leg thawed, he would be helpless. He lost his leg, but saved his life. And that's what will also happen to you. If you leave it frozen, you will lose the frozen part.

If a frozen foot has thawed and the patient must be transported, use cotton between toes (or fluff sterile gauze from the emergency kit and place between toes) and cover other areas with a loose bandage to protect the skin during sleeping bag stretcher evacuation. The use of Spenco 2nd Skin for blister care would be ideal, see page 216. If a fracture also exists, immobilize when in the field—loosely so as not to impair the circulation any further.

Cold-Induced Bronchospasm

Cold-induced bronchospasm, a form of asthma sometimes called "frozen lung" or pulmonary chilling, occurs when breathing rapidly at very low temperatures, generally below -20° F (-29° C). There is burning pain, sometimes coughing of blood, frequently asthmatic wheezing and, with irritation of the diaphragm, pain in the shoulder(s) and upper stomach that may last for 1 to 2 weeks. The treatment is bedrest, steam inhalations, drinking extra water, humidification of the living area, and no smoking. Avoid this condition by using parka hoods, face masks, or breathing through mufflers, which result in re-breathing the warmed, humidified, expired air.

Immersion Foot

Immersion foot results from wet, cool conditions with temperature exposures from 68° F (20° C) down to freezing. This is an extremely serious injury that can be worse than frostbite. There are two stages of this problem. In the first stage the foot is cold, swollen, waxy, and mottled with dark burgundy to blue splotches. This foot is resilient to palpation, whereas the frozen foot is very hard. Skin is sodden and friable. Loss of feeling makes walking difficult. The second stage lasts from days to weeks. The feet are swollen, red, and hot; blisters form; infection and gangrene are common.

To prevent this problem, avoid nonbreathing (rubber) footwear when possible, dry the feet and change wool socks when feet get wet or sweaty (certainly every night), periodically elevate, air, dry, and massage the feet to promote circulation. Avoid tight, constricting clothing. As a minimum, remove boots and socks nightly, drying the feet and warming them before sleeping.

Treatment differs from frostbite and hypothermia in the following ways: (1) Give the patient 10 grains (650 mg) of aspirin every 6 hours to help decrease platelet adhesion and clotting ability of the blood; (2) give additional Lorcet 10/650 every 4 hours for pain, but discontinue as soon as possible; (3) provide 1 ounce of hard liquor (30 mL) every hour while awake and 2 ounces (60 mL) every 2 hours during sleeping hours to vasodilate or increase the flow of blood to the feet. If you are unsure whether or not you are dealing with immersion foot or frostbite, or if you may have suffered both, treat for frostbite.

Chilblains

Chilblains result from exposure of dry skin to temperatures from 60° F (16° C) to freezing. The skin is red, swollen, frequently tender, and itching. This is the mildest form of cold injury and no tissue loss results. Treatment is the prevention of further exposure with protective clothing over bare skin and the use of ointments if available, such as A & D Ointment or Vaseline (white petrolatum). The hydrocortisone 1% cream from the Topical Bandaging Module will help when applied 4 times daily.

Heat-Stress Injuries

High environmental temperatures are frequently aggravated by strenuous work; humidity; reflection of heat from rock, sand, or other structures (even snow!); and the lack of air movement. It takes a human approximately 10 days to become heat acclimated. Once heat stress adaptation takes place, there will be a decrease in the loss of salt in the sweat produced, to conserve electrolytes. Another major change is the rapid production of sweat and the formation of larger quantities of sweat. Thus the body is able to start its efficient cooling mechanism—sweating—more fully and with less electrolyte disturbance to the body.

Salt lost in sweat during work can normally be replaced at mealtime. An unacclimatized man working an 8-hour shift would sweat 4 to 6 liters of sweat. The salt content is high, namely 3 to 5 gram/liter of sweat. With acclimatization, salt concentration drops (1 to 2 gram/liter). Thus an acclimatized man might lose 6 to 16 grams of salt during an 8-hour shift in 6 to 8 liters of sweat. The unacclimatized man could lose a total of 18 to 30 grams of salt in 4 to 6 liters of sweat. The average American diet contains 10 to 15 grams/day of salt. This means that an unacclimatized worker could be suffering from a 3- to 20-gram salt deficit per day. In the 10 days that it would take his body to become conditioned to heat stress, the total salt deficit could become substantial.

A concern in heat illness prevention is that a heat-stressed individual must obtain adequate fluid replacement. If we focus on salt replacement, to the exclusion of adequate water intake, the individual may become salt loaded and accelerate his dehydration. Generally, an excess of salt or water over actual needs is readily controlled by kidney excretion.

Depletion of body salt *can* lead to progressive dehydration because the body will attempt to maintain a balance between electrolyte concentration in tissue fluids with that in the cells. Deficient salt intake, with continued intake of water, tends to dilute tissue fluid. This suppresses the antidiuretic hormone (ADH) of the pituitary gland, preventing the kidney from reabsorbing water. The kidney will then excrete a large volume of very dilute urine. The salt concentration of body fluids will be maintained, but at the cost of increasing the depletion of body water with a rapid onset of dehydration. Under heat stress, this can result in symptoms of heat exhaustion similar to those resulting from water restriction, but with more severe signs of circulatory insufficiency and notably little thirst. Absence of chloride in the urine (less than 3 gm/liter) is diagnostic of salt deficiency.

The ideal replacement fluid for the unacclimatized worker would be lightly salted water (0.1% or 1 tsp/gal, 1 gram/liter), to prevent water or salt depletion. He will need 13 to 20 ounces (400 to 600 ml) of water before activity and 3 to 6 ounces (90 to 180 ml) of water every 10 to 15 minutes during an active period. Do not go longer than 30 minutes between drinks of water. Replacement fluids should not contain greater sugar concentrations than 6 grams per 100 ml of water, as these higher concentrations slow gastric emptying. Acclimatized subjects will need only water as a replacement fluid, but will need 32 ounces (1 liter) per hour. Thirst may lag behind requirements, so that oral replacement should be voluntarily done before thirst even becomes noticeable. Water deprivation is dangerous and can be avoided.

With no water available, how long could a person expect to survive? The answer is generally dependent upon the temperature and the amount of activity. At a temperature of 120° F (49° C) with no water available, the victim would expect to survive about 2 days (regardless of activity). This temperature is so high that survival would not be increased beyond 2 days by even 4 quarts (3.7 l) of water. Ten quarts (9.5 l) might provide an extra day. At 90° F (32° C) with no water, the person could survive about 5 days if she walked during the day, 7 days if travel was only at night or if no travel was undertaken at all. With 4 quarts of water, survival would extend to 6.5 days with day travel and to 10 days with only night travel. With 10 quarts, days of survival would increase to 8 and 15 respectively. If the highest temperature was 60° (15.5° C) with no water, the active person could expect to survive 8 days, the inactive person 10 days.

Heat Cramps

Salt depletion can result in nausea, twitching of muscle groups, and at times severe cramping of abdominal muscles, legs, or elsewhere.

Treatment of *heat cramps* consists of stretching the muscles involved (avoid aggressive massage), resting in a cool environment, and replacing salt losses. Generally 10 to 15 grams of salt and generous water replacement should be adequate treatment.

Heat Exhaustion

Heat exhaustion is a classic example of compensatory shock (see page 15), encountered while working in a hot environment. The body has dilated the blood vessels in the skin to divert heat from the core to surface for cooling. However this dilation is so pronounced, coupled with profuse sweating and loss of fluid (also a part of the cooling process) that the blood pressure to the entire system falls too low to adequately supply the brain and the visceral organs. The patient will have a rapid heartrate and other findings associated with the compensatory stage of shock: pale color, nausea, dizziness, headache, and a light-headed feeling. Generally the patient is sweating profusely, but this may not always be the case. The temperature may be elevated.

Treat as for shock. Have the patient lie down immediately, elevate the feet to increase the blood supply to the head, remove from direct sunlight and the hot environment. Provide copious amounts of water, a minimum of 1 to 2 quarts. Lightly salted water would be best. Obviously, fluids can only be administered if the patient is conscious. If unconscious, elevate the feet 3 feet above head level and protect from aspiration of vomit. Give water when the patient awakens.

Heat Stroke

Heat stroke (sun stroke) represents the complete breakdown of the heat control process (thermal regulation) in the human body. With the loss of the ability to sweat, core temperatures rise over 105° F (40° C) rapidly and soon exceed 107.6° F (42° C), resulting in death if not treated aggressively. THIS IS A TRUE EMERGENCY. It is a progressive stage of shock. The patient will be confused, very belligerent and uncooperative, and rapidly become unconscious. Immediately move into shade or erect a hasty barrier for shade. Spray with water or other suitable fluid and fan vigorously to lower the core temperature through evaporative cooling. This is the one time in medicine when it may be justifiable to urinate on your patient. Massage limbs to allow the cooler blood of the extremities to return to core circulation more readily and fan to increase evaporative heat loss. Carefully monitor the core temperature and cease cooling when it lowers to 102° F (39° C). The temperature may continue to fall or suddenly raise again.

The most significant finding in heat stroke is the *altered mental status* of the victim. While heat exhaustion victims can be confused, this should resolve rapidly when they are in the shock treatment position (head down, feet up). The confusion and very often belligerent behavior of heat stroke victims make them very hard to handle. While their skin is normally dry and hot, this is not always the case. Suspect heat stroke in anyone who becomes confused and erratic in behavior, or unconscious, during exercise in a hot environment.

This person should be evacuated as soon as possible since his thermal regulation mechanism is quite unstable and will remain so for an undeterminable length of time. He should be placed under a physician's care as soon as possible. Terminate the expedition, if necessary, to evacuate.

Prickly Heat

Prickly heat is a heat rash caused by the entrapment of sweat in glands in the skin. This can result in skin irritation and frequently severe itching. Treatment includes cooling and drying the involved area and avoiding conditions that may induce sweating for a while. Providing several hours of cool, dry environment daily is the only reliable treatment for prickly heat, but you may treat for itch as indicated on page 32.

Lightning

Other than being totally toasted, cardiopulmonary arrest is the most significant lightning injury. People who can scream from fright or pain after an electrical bolt has struck are already out of immediate danger. Their wounds may be dressed later. Those who appear dead must have immediate attention as they may be saved. Normally when dealing with mass casualties the wounded are cared for preferentially, while the dead are left alone. Not in this instance! The victim is highly unlikely to die unless cardiopulmonary arrest occurs. But if cardiopulmonary arrest does happen, 75% will die unless CPR is performed. As the heart tends to restart itself due to its inherent ability (automaticity), the heartbeat may return spontaneously in a short time. The respiratory system, however, may be shut down for 5 to 6 hours before being able to resume its normal rhythm. Lack of oxygen will cause a person whose heart has restarted spontaneously to die. When administrating CPR, take precautions with the cervical spine as the explosion may have caused fractures of the neck or other portions of the body. While CPR is being performed, check for the pulse periodically. When the heart restarts, maintain ventilations for the patient until respirations also resume. Attempt to continue this as long as possible; a victim may be revived even after many hours with no neurological defects—but only if CPR or respiration ventilation has been properly performed. Remember, after a lightning strike the victim's eyes may be fixed and dilated, respirations ceased, heart stopped, blood pressure 0/0—all signs of clinical death. Pay no attention to these findings, but administer CPR as long as physically possible.

Lightning frequently causes vascular spasms in its victim. This can result in faint, or even non-palpable pulses. When the vasospasm clears, which it generally does within a few hours, the pulses return.

Neurological defects are the second major consequence of lightning hits. Approximately 72% of victims suffer loss of consciousness and three-quarters of these people will have a cardiopulmonary arrest. Direct damage to the brain can result, but frequently the neurological defects, to include seizure activity and abnormal brainwave studies, eventually revert to normal. Two-thirds of victims will have neurological defects of the lower half of their bodies, one-third will suffer from paralysis of the upper half. Amnesia and confusion of events after the accident are common, but usually transient.

Most will have amnesia, confusion, and short-term memory loss that may last 2 to 5 days. These effects are similar to those experienced by electroconvulsive shock therapy patients. The person may be able to talk intelligently, but shortly thereafter not remember the conversation had taken place.

Burns from the lightning itself are generally not severe. Very high voltage is carried over the surface of conductors. The high voltage of lightning is similarly carried over the surface of the body with minimal internal burn damage, the so-called *flashover effect*.

Direct electrical burn damage can occur, however, and when it does it usually consists of one of several types: *Linear burns* start at the head, progress down the chest, and split to continue down both legs. These burns are usually ½ to 1½ inches in width and are first and second degree. They follow areas of heavy sweat concentration. *Punctate burns* look like a buckshot wound. These are full thickness, third-degree burns that are discrete, round wounds, measuring from a few millimeters to a centimeter in width. These seldom require grafting as the area is so small. *Feathering or ferning burns* are diagnostic of lightning injury. They fade within a few hours to days and require no treatment. This phenomenon is not a true burn, but the effect of electron showers on the skin. They have a characteristic reddish fern appearance that covers the skin surface—especially the trunk. *Thermal burns* also result from vaporization of surface moisture, combustion of clothing, heated metal buckles, etc. Thermal burns are the most common type of lightning-associated burn and they can be first-, second-, or third-degree.

The flash-over effect saves most victims from burn trauma. However, as noted, burns do occur. Persons with head burns are two and a half times more likely to die than those without. Possibly more surprising, persons with leg burns are five times more likely to die than those who do not have them. This is probably related to a ground or step current phenomenon.

The four mechanisms of direct lightning injury are: (1) direct strike,

(2) splash, (3) step current, (4) blunt trauma. To minimize the chance of lightning injury, the following should be noted about these mechanisms:

1. *Direct strikes* are most likely to take place in the open, especially if carrying metal or objects above shoulder level. Shelter should be taken within the *cone of safety,* described as a 45° angle down from a tall object, such as a tree or cliff face.

2. *Splash injuries* are perhaps the most common mechanism of lightning hit—the current strikes a tree or other object and jumps to a person whose body has less resistance than the object the lightning initially struck. Splash injuries may occur from person to person, when several people are standing close together. It has jumped from fences after having struck the fence some distance away. It has splashed to people from plumbing fixtures inside houses that were struck. Avoid close proximity to walls, fences, plumbing, or other items that could be struck.

3. *Step current* is also called stride voltage and ground current. The lightning current spreads out in a wave along the ground from the struck object, with the current strength decreasing as the radius from the strike increases. If the victim's feet are at different distances from the point of the strike, and the resistance in the ground greater than through his body, he will complete a circuit. Large groups of people can be injured simultaneously in this manner. Keeping feet and legs together, while squatting down, minimizes the chances of step voltage injury.

4. *Blunt trauma,* or the sledge-hammer effect, results from the force of the lightning strike, or the explosive shock wave that it produces. The victim may be forcibly knocked to the ground. Over 50% of victims will have their eardrums ruptured in one or both ears. This may result from direct thermal damage, the thunder shock wave, or even skull fractures from the blunt trauma. Barotrauma to the ears may be reduced by keeping the mouth open during times of great danger.

In the above scenario a person should squat, with legs together and mouth open in a zone of safety—but not too near the protective tree or cliff face. Spread party members out to maximize the chance that there will be survivors, and thus rescuers, if lightning strikes appear imminent. Get boats into a zone of safety near shore against the tree line or cliff face. Other than the immediate presence of lightning, is there any warning? At times there will be the smell of ozone, hair may stand on end, metal climbing equipment may start to vibrate, or St. Elmo's fire may be present. Good luck!

High Altitude Illnesses

High-altitude–related illnesses can generally be avoided by *gradual* exposure to higher elevation, with the camping or sleeping ascent rate not exceeding 1,000 feet (300 meters) per day when above 9,000 feet (2,800 meters). Alternatively, avoid sleeping at greater than 2,000 foot (600 meter) increments every 2 days when suddenly traveling from near sea level to 10,000 feet (3000 meters).

A high carbohydrate diet, consisting of at least 70 percent carbohydrates started 1 to 2 days prior to ascent, remaining well hydrated, and exercising moderately until altitude acclimatized, all help prevent high altitude illness.

The three major clinical manifestations of this disease complex are acute mountain sickness (AMS), high altitude pulmonary edema (HAPE), and high altitude cerebral edema (HACE). As will be noted, the symptoms progress rather insidiously. They are not clear-cut, separate diseases—they often occur together. The essential therapy for each of them is *recognition and descent*. This is life-saving and more valuable than the administration of oxygen or drugs. To prevent high altitude illnesses it is helpful to "climb high, but camp low,"—that is, spend nights at the lowest camp elevation feasible. More information on high altitude illnesses can be found at my Web site.

Acute Mountain Sickness (AMS)

Rarely encountered below 6,500 feet (2,000 meters), acute mountain sickness (AMS) is common in persons going above 10,000 feet (3,000 meters) without taking the time to acclimatize for altitude. Symptoms beginning soon after ascent consist of headache (often severe), nausea, vomiting, shortness of breath, weakness, sleep disturbance, and occasionally a periodic breathing known to medical personnel as Cheyne-Stokes breathing.

Prevention, as with all of the high altitude illnesses, is gradual ascent above 9,000 (2,800 meters) feet and light physical activity for the first several days. For persons especially prone to AMS, it may be helpful to take acetazolamide (Diamox) prophylactically 125 mg every 12 hours starting the day of ascent and continuing the next 3 to 5 days. This medication helps prevent or treat the acid-base imbalance of the blood that can occur in some people from the increased loss of carbon dioxide at high altitudes. The treatment dose of acetazolamide is 250 mg twice daily for 5 days. This prescription drug should be added to your medical kit if you expect to encounter elevations above 9,000 feet. See Diamox, page 225.

The best AMS treatment is descent, and relief can often be felt even if the descent is only 2,000 to 3,000 feet (600 to 900 meters). Full relief can be obtained by descending to below 6,500 feet (2,000 meters). Stricken individuals should avoid heavy exercise, but sleep does not help as breathing is slower during sleep making oxygen deprivation worse. Oxygen will only help if taken continuously for 12 to 48 hours. Aspirin may be used for headache. Percogesic or ibuprofen from the Non-Rx Oral Medication Module may be used. In addition to descent, Decadron (dexamethasone) 4 mg tablets every 6 hours until below the altitude at which symptoms appeared has been shown to help control the symptoms of AMS. Decadron tablets or injection should be added to your medical kit if you expect to encounter elevations above 10,000 feet. See Decadron, pages 225 and 227. Also see headache, page 34.

High Altitude Pulmonary Edema (HAPE)

High altitude pulmonary edema (HAPE) is rare below 8,000 feet (2,500 meters), but occurs at higher altitude in those poorly acclimatized. It is more likely in persons between the ages of 5 and 18 (the incidence is apparently less than 0.4% in persons over 21 and as high as 6% in those younger); in those who have had this problem before; and in those who have been altitude acclimatized and who are returning to high altitude after spending approximately 2 weeks at sea level.

Prevention is altitude acclimatization as discussed in the section on AMS above. Nifedipine (Procardia) 20 mg every 8 hours to be taken during the ascent phase and for 3 additional days at altitude has been shown to work prophylactically.

Symptoms develop slowly within 24 to 60 hours of arrival at high altitude with shortness of breath, irritating cough, weakness, rapid heart rate, and headache that rapidly progress to intractable cough with bloody sputum, low-grade fever, and increasing chest congestion. Symptoms may progress profoundly at night. Climbers should be evaluated by listening to their chests for a fine crackling sound (called *rales*) and resting pulse rate checked nightly. A pulse rate of greater than 110 per minute or respirations greater than 16 per minute after a 20 minute rest is an early sign of HAPE. Respirations over 20 per minute and pulse over 130 per minute indicates a medical emergency and the patient must be evacuated immediately. Without treatment, death usually occurs within 6 to 12 hours after onset of coma.

Descent to lower altitude is essential and should not be delayed. Treatment includes nifedipine 20 mg sublingual (or chewed and swallowed) given upon diagnosis and repeated every 6 hours. Oxygen may be of value if given continuously over the next 12 to 48 hours, starting at 6 liters/minute for the first 15 minutes, then reduced to 2 liters/minute. A snug face mask is better than nasal prongs. Oxygen may provide rapid relief in mild cases, however it should be continued for a minimum of 6 to 12 hours, if possible. Oxygen is not a substitute for descent in severe cases. A descent of as little as 2,000 to 3,000 feet (600 to 900 meters) may result in prompt improvement. The portable hyperbaric chamber called a Gamow Bag is very useful in reversing the effects of high altitude; (see Figure 7-1). When zipped shut with the patient inside, this nylon bag is pressurized with the use of a foot or mechanical pump. A difference of 1½ pounds per square inch is formed when the bag is fully pressurized, resulting in a significant apparent decrease in altitude for the patient (see Table 7-1). Length of treatment time in the bag would be

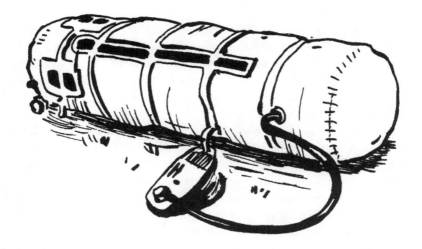

Figure 7-1: Gamow Bag used for simulating descent in the treatment of the high altitude illnesses.

until symptoms cleared and the climbing conditions permit the aided descent of the patient.

High Altitude Cerebral Edema (HACE)

High altitude cerebral edema (HACE) is less common than AMS or HAPE, but it is more dangerous. Death has occurred from HACE at altitude as low as 8,000 feet (2,500 meters); however HACE is rare below 11,500 feet (3,500 meters). The symptoms are increasingly severe headache, mental confusion, emotional behavior, hallucinations, unstable gait, loss of vision, loss of dexterity, and facial muscle paralysis. The victim may fall into a restless sleep, followed by a deep coma and death.

Descent is essential. The use of the Gamow Bag, as indicated above, can be life-saving. Oxygen should be administered starting at 6 liters/minute for the first 15 minutes, followed by a flow rate of 2 liters/minute. Decadron (dexamethasone) should be given in large doses, namely 10 mg intravenously, followed by 4 mg every 6 hours intramuscularly until the symptoms subside. Response is usually noted within 12 to 24 hours and the dosage may be reduced after 2 to 4 days and gradually discontinued over a period of 5 to 7 days. Immediate descent and oxygen are recommended to prevent permanent neurological damage or death.

Other High Altitude Conditions

Generalized swelling of the face, arms, and legs can appear after arrival at high altitude and may persist for days or even weeks. It is more common in women than men. The cause is unknown and no treatment is required. The swelling disappears after descent. The use of diuretics to eliminate this problem should be discouraged as they can lead to increased problems with dehydration.

Hemorrhages of the retinal blood vessels (of the eye) can occur at altitudes over 14,000 feet (4,300 meters) and are frequently found in climbers over 17,600 feet (5,365 meters). This condition rarely causes visual difficulty. There is no treatment. It resolves several weeks after return to sea level. Increased flatulence may be noted in high altitude, a condition referred to in the medical journals as HAFE (high altitude flatulent expulsion). Foods known to cause gas at lower altitude should be avoided. Simethicone products can be taken to help control this problem, such as Phazyme 125, 1 tablet with meals and at bedtime. This medication is available without a prescription. (Several medical journals decline publishing any further articles on this topic. Of the many already published, not much substance can be found, so they are considered to be more or less hot air.)

High altitude cachexia (HAC) is the name that has been given to the extreme weight loss that climbers note on long, high altitude climbs above 17,000 feet (5,200 meters). Providing adequate amounts of carbohydrate seems to curtail some muscle loss. Fats and proteins become less palatable at high altitude. Climbers need between 5,000 and 6,000 kcal/day: 55% from carbohydrates, 35% from fats, and 10% from proteins.

Dehydration is a significant problem from respiratory loss in the cold, dry air and due to rapid breathing rates. Climbers become dehydrated, yet frequently urinate a dilute urine, rather than concentrating and conserving body fluid as is usual under dehydration circumstances.

Vitamin intake should be approximately 3 times the recommended daily allowances due to the high calorie intake. To consume 6,000 kcal/day, a person would have to be in excellent physical shape. Most healthy young people cannot use more than 4,200 kcal/day, yet I have encountered wilderness brutes who required 8,000 kcal/day for weeks on end. Be sure that the cook's larder is ready for them or they can become very unhappy campers.

Sawyer® Accident/Evacuation Record

Patient Name _____ Age _____ Sex _____

Date/Time of Accident _____

Weather: Temp _____ Rain/Snow _____ Visibility _____ Wind _____
(mph)

Type of illness or injury: _____

Is patient on medication/drugs? _____

Physical Examination Findings: _____

_____

_____

Can patient eat, drink? _____ Last food intake _____ Allergies _____

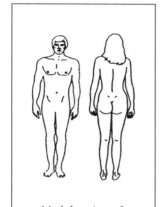

Mark location of
injuries or pain

Primary Survey: Survey the scene for additional hazards; check the airway; check circulation; protect the neck.

Secondary Survey: *Head*–look for wounds, fluid coming from eyes, nose, ears, mouth, check level of consciousness (alert, only responds to verbal, only responds to pain, or unresponsive).

Neck–is airway OK, pain along spine to touch

Chest–compress ribs from side, any pain or deformity

Abdomen–press gently, any spasm, distension, pain

Back–touch along the spine, note point tenderness

Pelvis–cup crest of hip and press gently downward toward midline of body looking for instability or pain

Legs–squeeze each one from groin to toes looking for lack of circulation, sensation, or motion in toes

We require (tents, clothing, medical supplies, food) _____

_____

_____

Our location is: _____

Our plan is to: _____

On the reverse indicate medical experience/training/number of party members who can help, days of food on hand. Draw a map of location or intended route.

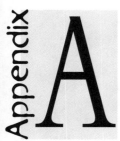

The Wilderness Expedition Medical Kit

While it is possible to improvise to a great extent, an appropriate first aid kit is one of the ten basic essentials that should be brought on any wilderness outing. The most compact kit will also be the one that contains both multifunctional and crossfunctional components. This requires the minimal number of medications, but provides in-depth coverage when a particular medication is consumed.

Taking the above into account, study the actual first aid material requirements encountered by others on similar trips, anticipate the most likely serious events that could conceivably occur, and tailor the kit to the medical skill level of the participants. Additional factors to consider are the weight, cost, bulk, and availability of components. Take into consideration the number in the party, length of trip, degree of risk anticipated, and whether or not other people beyond those of the immediate party will be treated.

If you are designing a commercial kit, two additional factors must also considered. One is what real estate agents call "curb appeal." It has to look impressive at first glance. The other is to plan for various price points to target different markets. These constraints give commercial kits a disadvantage over the kit you put together yourself. Sources for kit components can be found at the Web site at www.adventure-media.com/wildernessmedicine5/. The ten basic kit essentials are also displayed at that site.

Most injuries and conditions described in this book can be treated with very little in the way of kit components. But I have included here state-of-the-art items that would provide ideal treatment aid. As this book has been written for those who may be isolated without ready access to professional medical care, the treatments discussed go beyond normal first aid. The kit described in this Appendix similarly goes beyond what would be considered a "first aid" kit, but the initial modules are indeed easily useable under first aid conditions. The kit consists of 4 units: Topical Bandaging Module, Non-Rx Oral Medication Module, Rx Oral/Topical Medication Module, and the Rx Injectable Medication Module.

As a minimum, the Topical Bandaging Module and Non-Rx Oral Medication Module will generally fulfill the vast majority of emergency treatment requirements. The prescription modules are designed for long-term, and more advanced, patient care. All items listed in the kit modules can be obtained without a prescription, except in the modules clearly marked "Rx."

All nonprescription medications have packaging that describes the official dosages and appropriate warnings or precautions concerning their use. Prescription medications usually have elaborate package inserts with this same information. When obtaining a prescription drug for your medical kit, request this insert from your physician or copy the information from the Physicians' Desk Reference (PDR), which is available at libraries and bookstores everywhere.

 Brand Names have been used to simplify spelling and product recognition or to minimize potential confusion between similar sounding and variations in generic names between American, Canadian, and British sources.

 Alternative Improvisation. Alternatives to the use of these various medications are discussed in the treatment discussions for various problems throughout the book. Alternatives to various medical supplies are discussed below.

Topical Bandaging Module

Quantity	Item
10 pkg	Spyroflex® 2" x 2" wound dressings (or carry 2 for each person)
2 pkg	Spenco 2nd Skin® Burn Dressing Kits (or carry 1 for 2 people)
15 pkg	Nu-Gauze®, high absorbent, sterile, 2 ply, 3" x 3v, pkg/2
25	Coverlet® Bandage Strips 1" x 3"
1	Tape, Waterproof 1" x 15'
1	Sam Splint® 36"
1	Elastic Bandage 3"
1	Elastic Bandage 4"
1	Max Strength Triple Antibiotic Ointment with pramoxine, 1 oz tube
1	Hibiclens® surgical scrub, 4 oz bottle
1	Tetrahydrozoline Ophthalmic Drops, 0.05%, 15 ml bottle
1	Hydrocortisone cream 1%, 1 oz tube
1	Clotrimazole cream, 2%, ½ oz tube
1	Cavit® dental filling paste
2 pair	Examination gloves
1	Irrigation syringe
1	Sawyer Extractor®
1	Surgical kit consisting of 1 needle holder, 2 each 3-0 ethicon sutures, 1 each 5-0 ethicon suture, and 2 each 3-0 gut sutures
1	Over-pack container for above

Spyroflex® 2" x 2" wound dressings.

Made by PolyMedica Industries, Spyroflex is a multi-use bandaging system that replaces wound closure strips *and* coverings. It accelerates blood clotting, holds lacerations closed, protects the wound from the outside, treats abraded skin as well as leaking and dry wounds, and is an excellent cover for first and second degree burns. Most importantly, it establishes a local environment that speeds up wound healing. The dressing is a "smart" dressing that absorbs and evaporates the correct amount of vapor to produce the proper healing condition. This dressing can be left in place for up to 10 days, thus decreasing the need for large quantities of bulky dressings.

 Cellophane and duct tape: cellophane, plastic food wrappers, or plastic sheeting of any kind makes an excellent wound covering. Held down with tape of any type, a cellophane dressing is non-adherent, seepage leaks from the unsealed edges, the wound can be observed, and the increased and appropriate moisture level of the dressing increases the rate of wound healing.

Spenco 2nd Skin®

Truly a major advance in field medicine. This inert hydrogel consists of 96% water and 4% polyethylene oxide. It is used on wet, weeping wounds to absorb fluids and protect the injury. This is a perfect prevention or cure for friction blisters. It revolutionized the field treatment of first-, second-, and third-degree burns, as it can be applied to all three as a covering and for pain relief. This item should be in every medical kit. The ideal covering pad is the Spenco Adhesive Knit Bandage. If used in treating blisters, remove only the outer covering of cellophane from the 2nd Skin, cover with the Knit Bandage, and occasionally dampen with clean water to maintain the hydrogel's hydration. It will last a lot longer this way when in short supply.

 Cooling technique for burns (see page 107), piece of tape over hot spots (see page 106).

Nu-Gauze® Pads

J&J Company has developed a gauze that is 2 ply yet absorbs nearly 50% more fluid than conventional 12-ply gauze pads. This may not seem important until a rapidly bleeding wound needs care. For years J&J has made a "Nu-Gauze" strip packing dressing; the Nu-Gauze Pads are a completely different material. They are a wonderful advance in gauze design.

 Cotton t-shirts or other clothing, bandannas.

Coverlet Bandage Strips

A Beiersdorf product, these common 1" x 3" bandage strips are the best made. They stick even when wet, will last through days of hard usage, and stretch for compression on a wound and conform for better application.

 Duct tape, climbing tape.

Waterproof Tape

A tough tape that can be used for splinting or bandage application. There are no brand advantages that I can determine. A 1" by 15' roll on a metal spool is a useable size.

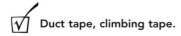 Duct tape, climbing tape.

Sam Splint®

A padded, malleable splint that provides enough comfort to be used as a neck collar. It is adequately rigid to splint any extremity and universal so that only one of these need be carried for all splinting needs. This item replaces ladder splints, etc. I never recommended the inclusion of splints in wilderness medical kits until this product was developed. It weighs less than 5 ounces.

 Malleable splints can frequently be made from stays found in internal backpack frames. Other stiff materials can be used such as strips of ensolite foam pads or inflatable pads, held in place with tape or torn cloth.

Elastic Bandage, 2"   Obtain good quality bandages that stretch without narrowing and which
Elastic Bandage, 3"   provide firm, consistent compression.
Elastic Bandage, 6"

 Elastic bandages can be replaced with almost any cloth that is firmly wrapped in place. The most stretchy form of cloth usually available is a cotton t-shirt.

Maximum Strength Triple Antibiotic Ointment with pramoxine, 1 oz tube

Each gram of this ointment contains bacitracin 500 units, neomycin sulfate 3.5 mg, polymyxin B sulfate 10,000 units, and an anesthetic pramoxine hydrochloride 10 mg. For use as a topical antibiotic in the prevention and treatment of minor infections of abrasions and burns. This formulation also is an anesthetic that numbs the skin. A light coat should be applied twice daily. Neomycin can cause skin rash and itch in some people. If this develops, discontinue use and apply the hydrocortisone cream to counter this effect.

 Honey or granulated sugar placed on wounds is painless and kills germs by dehydrating them. A strong sugar solution draws the fluid from the bacteria, but human cells are able to actively avoid the dehydration process and are not injured with this technique.

Hibiclens® Surgical Scrub

This Stuart product (chlorhexidine gluconate 4%) far surpasses hexa-chlorophene and povidone-iodine scrub in its antiseptic action. The onset and duration of its action is much more impressive than either of those two products.

 Many surgical scrubs are available without prescription and are ideal for wilderness use, but they can all be replaced with potable (drinkable) water irrigation. Remember, "the solution to pollution is dilution."

Tetrahydrozoline ophthalmic drops 0.05%, 15 ml bottle

These eyedrops are used for allergy relief, to remove redness, and to alleviate discomfort from smoke, eye strain, etc. They will not cure infection or disguise the existence of a foreign body. Place 1 or 2 drops in each eye every 6 hours.

 Rinse eyes with clean water. A wet, cold compress relieves eye itch and pain.

Hydrocortisone Cream 1%, 1 oz. tube

This non-Rx steroid cream treats allergic skin rashes, such as those from poison ivy. A cream is ideal for treating weeping lesions, as opposed to dry scaly ones, but will work on either. For best results, cover with an occlusive dressing (plastic cover) overnight.

 Blistery rashes can be soothed and the leaking fluid dried by applying a cloth made wet with concentrated salt solution.

Clotrimazole cream 2%, ½ oz tube

This is one of the most effective antifungal preparations available for foot, groin, or other body fungal infections. Brand names are Lotrimin® and Mycelex® (vaginal cream). The vaginal cream in a 2 ounce tube is less expensive and works well on the skin surface, as well as vaginally.

 Dry, itchy lesions of any type respond to a soothing coating of cooking oil.

Cavit® dental filling paste

For temporary filling of cavities and repair of broken bridge work. Without being able to drill out the underlying decay, the cavity will need to be seen as soon as possible by a dentist for proper care or an abscess may form.

 Use oil of cloves to line the cavity for pain relief. A mixture of zinc-oxide powder (not the ointment) and oil of cloves, made up as a thick paste, can also be used as a temporary filling.

Protective gloves

Due to concerns with blood-borne pathogens (hepatitis B, C and AIDS), it is prudent to carry protective gloves for first aid use. These can be non-sterile (they are readily sterilized by boiling or treating with antiseptics). Vinyl gloves will last much longer in a kit than latex gloves, but the best are nitril gloves.

 Use an empty food bag or waterproof stuff sack as a glove, or wrap your hand in the most waterproof material available.

Irrigation Syringe

Required for forceful irrigation of wounds. The best would have a protective spray shield, such as the Zero-Wet® shield; otherwise, wear glasses to protect your eyes from splash contamination.

 The solution to pollution is dilution. Forceful irrigation is the best method for cleaning a wound and diluting the germ count enough so that the body's immune system can kill the remaining germs. Without a syringe, augment the volume of water that you are pouring on the wound with a brisk scrubbing action using a soft, clean cloth.

Surgical kit

Consisting of 1 needle holder, 2 each 3-0 ethicon sutures, 1 each 5-0 ethicon suture, and 2 each 3-0 gut sutures.

 Use the Spyroflex wound dressing as a surface closure. Lacking other means of fastening gaping wounds together, use the technique of open packing the wound with a wet-to-dry dressing described on page 91.

Non-Rx Oral Medication Module

Quantity	Item
24	Percogesic® tablets (pain, fever, muscle spasm, sleep aid, anxiety, congestion)
24	Ibuprofen 200 mg tablets (pain, fever, bursitis, tendonitis, menstrual cramps)
24	Diphenhydramine 25 mg capsules (antihistamine, anti-anxiety, cough, muscle cramps, nausea, and motion sickness prevention)
10	Bisacodyl 5 mg tablets (constipation)
12	Loperamide 2 mg tablets (diarrhea)
24	Cimetidine 200 mg tablets (heartburn, certain allergic reactions)
1	Over-pack container for above

 Alternatives to the use of these medications are discussed in the treatment options throughout the book. Each medication is multi-functional and also has cross-therapeutic versatility. This means that each item can be used for more than one problem, and problems have more than one drug that can be used for treatment. This allows a minimal number of medications to be carried in, yet provides depth in coverage if one medication is in short supply.

Percogesic® tablets

Relieve pain, fever, and muscle spasm. Each tablet contains 325 mg of acetaminophen and 30 mg of phenyltoloxamine citrate. Ideal for injuries of joints and muscles, as well as aches from infections. Phenyltoloxamine is also a decongestant. It also induces drowsiness and can be used as a sleeping aid or to calm a hysterical person. These indications are not included on the packaging information. Dosage is generally 2 tablets every 4 hours as needed. One of the most useful non-Rx drugs obtainable.

Ibuprofen tablets 200 mg

Brand names are Advil®, Nuprin®, and others. Relieves pain, fever, menstrual cramps, and inflammation. Over-use syndromes such as bursitis and tendonitis are common in wilderness-related activities and this is an ideal treatment. The non-Rx dosage is 2 tablets, 4 times a day. Should be taken with food to prevent stomach irritation or heartburn. The Rx dosage is 4 tablets taken 4 times daily, a dose that may be necessary for severe inflammation.

Diphenhydramine capsules 25 mg

The brand name is Benadryl®; many variations are sold containing other ingredients than just the diphenhydramine. For antihistamine action, these capsules can be taken 1 or 2 every 6 hours. To use as a powerful cough suppresser, the dose is 1 capsule every 6 hours. For muscle spasm relief, 1 or 2 capsules at bedtime alone or in combination with 2 ibuprofen 200 mg tables. For nausea or motion sickness, 1 capsule every 6 hours as needed.

Bisacodyl 5 mg

This laxative works on the large bowel to form a soft stool within 6 to 10 hours. Use 1 tablet as needed.

Loperamide 2 mg

An anti-diarrheal with the brand name of Imodium®. Dosage for persons 12 or older is 2 tablets after the first loose bowel movement followed by 1 tablet after each subsequent loose bowel movement, but no more than 4 tablets a day for no more than 2 days. The prescription use of this medication is usually 2 tablets immediately and 2 with each loose stools up to a maximum of 8 per day. Follow the package instructions for children's dosages.

Cimetidine 200 mg

Brand name is Tagamet®. This medication suppresses acid formation. It may be used to treat certain allergic reactions. The non-Rx dosage is 2 tablets four times daily. Prescription use goes as high as 4 tablets four times daily for acid suppression.

Rx Oral/Topical Medication Module

Quantity	Item
20	Doxycycline 100 mg tablets (antibiotic)
12	Zithromax® 250 mg tablets (antibiotic)
16	Levaquin® 500 mg tablets (antibiotic)
2	Diflucan® 150 mg tablets (antifungal) (for a female trip participant and 1 additional pill for each additional female on trip)
24	Lorcet® 10/650 tablets (pain, cough)

Rx Oral/Topical Medication Module *con't*

Quantity	Item
24	Atarax® 25 mg tablets (nausea, anxiety, antihistamine, pain medication augmentation)
1	Topicort® 0.25% ointment, ½ oz tube (skin allergy)
1	Tobradex® ophthalmic drops, 2.5 ml (eye, ear antibiotic and anti-inflammatory)
1	Tetracaine ophthalmic solution 0.5%, ⅛ oz tube (eye, ear anesthetic)
1	Denavir® (penciclovir) cream 1%, 5 gm tube (antiviral, lip and mouth sores)
1	Stadol® Nasal Spray (severe pain)
*	Diamox® 250 mg tablets, 10 per person (acute mountain sickness prevention)
*	Decadron® 4 mg tablets (10 per trip—allergy) (16 per climber at high risk—acute mountain sickness)
*	Flagyl® 250 mg (16 capsules for trichomonas or giardia infection).
*	Larium® (mefloquin) 250 mg (malaria protection; 1 per each week in malarious zone, plus 5 additional for each person on the expedition)
*	Fansidar® (sulfadoxine and pyrimethamine) tablets (malaria presumptive treatment; 6 tablets per every 10 people).
*	Famvir® 125 mg (24 per person with history of *H. simplex* cold sores, especially if going to altitude or expecting significant ultraviolet light exposure)

Doxycycline

The generic name of an antibiotic that is useful in treating many travel-related diseases. The various sections of the text dealing with infections will indicate the proper dosage, normally 1 tablet twice daily. Not to be used in children 8 years or younger or during pregnancy. May cause skin sensitivity on exposure to sunlight, thus causing an exaggerated sunburn. This does not usually happen, but be cautious during your first sun exposure when on this product. Many people traveling in the tropics have used this antibiotic safely. Very useful in malaria prevention at a dose of 1 tablet daily. Common brand names are Vibramycin®, Vibra-tabs®, and Monodox®.

Zithromax® 250 mg tablets

This is the brand name of azithromycin, a broad spectrum antibiotic used to treat certain types of pneumonia, infected throats, skin infections, and venereal diseases due to *Chlamydia trachomatis* or *Neisseria gonorrhoeae* and genital ulcer disease in men due to *Haemophilus ducreyi* (chancroid). Dosage is unique in that this medication is started by taking 2 tablets at once, then 1 tablet each 24 hours afterwards for 4 additional doses. These 6 tablets result in a therapeutic blood level for the next 5 days, thus providing a total of 10 days of coverage.

Levaquin® 500 mg

A broad spectrum antibiotic of a group known as fluoroquinolones. This medication is useful in treating diarrhea and even organisms resistant to the above antibiotics. It is useful in treating sinus infections, bronchitis, pneumonia, skin infections and skin ulcers, complicated urinary tract and kidney infections. Avoid excessive sun exposure while on this medication. Avoid in persons under the age of 18 and during nursing and pregnancy. Drink extra water when on this medication. Do not take with antacid, vitamins containing minerals, and ibuprofen, otherwise it may be taken at meal times. Some people are made dizzy by this medication. There is a possibility that it might cause tendonitis and should be stopped if muscle pain or tendon inflammation results. While used to treat diarrhea, it may cause diarrhea and it may result in vaginal monilia infection.

Diflucan® 150 mg

One tablet of this medication is taken to eliminate vaginal yeast (candidiasis) infection. These infections are at greater risk after taking broad spectrum antibiotics as they can suppress normal, healthy bacteria in the vagina. Tropical conditions are also a risk factor in developing this condition. While this medication often reacts with other medication, none are included in the Wilderness Medical Kit, and short-term use of 1 pill will normally not be significant regardless. The most common side effects are headache, nausea, and cramping.

Lorcet® 10/650

The brand name of the combination of 650 mg of acetaminophen and 10 mg of hydrocodone, the principal use of the drug is in the relief of pain. Hydrocodone is a powerful cough suppressor and also useful in treating abdominal cramping and diarrhea. The dosage of 1 tablet every 6 hours will normally control a severe toothache. Maximum dosage is 6 tablets per day. It may be augmented with Atarax®—see below.

Atarax® 25 mg

A brand name of hydroxyzine hydrochloride (note also the listing under "Vistaril®" in the Rx Injectable Medication Module), these tablets have multiple uses. They are a very powerful antinausea agent, muscle relaxant, antihistamine, antianxiety agent, sleeping pill, and will potentiate a pain medication (make it work better). For sleep 50 mg at bedtime; for nausea 25 mg ever 4 to 6 hours; to potentiate pain medication, take a 25 mg tablet with each dose of the pain medication. This medication treats rashes of all types and has a drying effect on congestion. The injectable version, Vistaril®, has identical actions.

Topicort® (desoximetasone) ointment 0.25%

This Rx steroid ointment treats severe allergic skin rashes. Dosage is a thin coat twice daily. Occlusive dressings are not required when using this product. Should be used with caution over large body surface areas or on children. Use should be limited to 10 days or less, particularly in the latter cases.

Tobradex® ophthalmic drops 2.5 ml

This is a combination of a powerful antibiotic (tobramycin .3%) and a steroid (dexamthasone .1%). It can be used to treat infections or allergies in the eye (for which it was designed) or the ear. It can be instilled in either location 2 to 3 times daily. This medication can cause complications in case of viral infections of the eye (which are rare compared to bacterial infections and allergy conditions).

Tetracaine ophthalmic solution (drops), 15 ml bottle

Sterile solution for use in eye or ear to numb pain. Do not reapply to eye if pain returns without examining for foreign body very carefully. Try not to use repeatedly in the eye as over-use delays healing. Continued pain may also mean you have missed a foreign body. Do not use in ears if considerable drainage is present; an eardrum may have ruptured and if this medication gets into the middle ear through a hole in the eardrum, it will cause profound vertigo (dizziness).

Denavir (penciclovir) cream 1%, 2 gram tube.

An antiviral treatment that is a useful treatment for cold sores on the face and on the lips. While not approved for use inside the mouth, this product actually works well there and is not harmful if swallowed. This may be used at high altitude to prevent the cold sores caused by intense ultraviolet light. Apply every 2 hours during waking hours for 4 days.

Stadol®, nasal spray

This is a powerful pain medication (generic name butorphanol) formulated to be absorbed by the lining of the nose. It is five times stronger than morphine on a milligram to milligram basis. Use only one spray up a nostril and wait 60 to 90 minutes before using a second spray in the other nostril. This process may be repeated in 3 to 4 hours. It should be working effectively within 20 minutes after the first spray. Over-spraying or allowing the medication to drain down the throat will waste it since it is inactivated by gastric fluids.

Diamox® 250 mg tablets

The brand name of acetazolamide, it is used in the prevention of acute mountain sickness for those contemplating rapid ascent to elevations over 9,000 feet. Side effects include tingling of the mouth and fingers, numbness, loss of appetite, and occasional instances of drowsiness and confusion—all signs of the acute mountain sickness that one is trying to prevent. Increased urination and rare sun sensitive skin rash is encountered. See text, page 207.

Decadron® (dexamethasone) 4 mg

For allergy ½ tablet twice daily after meals for 5 days. For treatment of acute mountain sickness give 4 mg every 6 hours until well below the altitude at which symptoms appeared. See text, pages 208 and 210.

Flagyl® 250 mg

The brand name of metronidazole, this antibiotic is useful in treating diarrhea caused by giardia (see page 177) at a dose of 250 mg 3 times daily. It is also used in treating infections by *Entamoeba histolytica* and *Trichomonas vaginalis* (both protozoal parasites) and certain other bacteria. May cause numbness and nausea. Should not be taken by people with central nervous system diseases. Do not drink alcohol with this drug as it causes flushing and vomiting.

Lariam® (mefloquine) 250 mg

Used to prevent malaria.

Fansidar®

The brand name of a tablet containing two medications—sulfadoxine and pyrimethamine—it can be taken 3 tablets at one time in the presumptive treatment of malaria. Immediately follow with evacuation of the patient for further treatment. Do not give to persons allergic to sulfa drugs, with liver or kidney disorders, or pregnant or nursing mothers. Bringing six tablets for every 10 people on a trip in a malarial region is adequate.

Famvir® 125 mg

This may be taken 3 times daily as prophylaxis to prevent *Herpes simplex* lip lesions, which are often activated by high altitude or reflective ultraviolet light exposure. Should be included in the kit if persons are known to have recurrent problems. An alternative is to use the Danvir cream.

Rx Injectable Medication Module

Quantity	Item
1	Nubain® 20 mg/ml, 10 ml multi-use vial (pain)
1	Lidocaine 1% 10 ml multi-use vial (local anesthetic)
6	3½ml syringes with 25 gauge, ⅝ inch needles
1+	Decadron® 4 mg/ml, 5 ml multi-use vial (steroid), 1 per trip for allergy; 3 vials per climber at risk for acute mountain sickness
3–6	Rocephin®, 500 gm vials (antibiotic)
1	Vistaril® 50 mg/ml, 10 ml multi-use vial (many uses)
2	Anakit® or AnaGuard® (bee stings—anaphylactic shock, asthma)

Nubain® (nalbuphine) 20 mg/ml, 10 ml vial

A strong, synthetic narcotic analgesic, it is available only by prescription but it is not a controlled narcotic. It is equal to morphine in strength. Normal adult dose is 10 mg (1/2 ml) given intramuscularly every 3 to 6 hours. The maximum dose is 20 mg (1 ml) every 3 hours.

Can be mixed with 25 to 50 mg of Vistaril® in the same syringe for increased analgesia in severe pain problems.

Lidocaine 1%

Injection for numbing wounds. Maximum amount to be used in a wound in an adult should be 15 ml. This fluid is also used to mix the Rocephin®. See the package insert that comes with the Rocephin®.

Syringes

Many types are available, but for wilderness use I find the 3½ml with the attached 25 gauge, ⅝ inch needle to be the most universally useful.

Decadron® (dexamethasone) 4 mg/ml

For use in allergic reactions, give 4 mg daily for 5 days IM. For Acute Mountain Sickness give 4 mg (1 ml) every 6 hours until well below the altitude where symptoms started. See pages 208 and 210.

Rocephin® (ceftriaxone) 500 mg vials

A broad spectrum antibiotic of the cephalosporin class, the injectable medication has a wide range of bactericidal activities, including pneumonia and bronchitis, skin infections, urinary tract and kidney infections, gonorrhea, pelvic infection, bone and joint infections, and intra-abdominal infections, and some types of meningitis. Each vial will require 0.9 ml of lidocaine 1% to mix the contents. The reconstituted medication is stable at room temperatures for 3 days.

Vistaril® 50mg/ml

A brand name of hydroxyzine hydrochloride, uses and dosages are the same as indicated for "Atarax®" in the Rx Oral/Topical Medication Module. Obviously in the treatment of profound vomiting, injections of medication will work better than oral administration. This solution can be mixed in the same syringe as the Nubain® for administration as one injection.

Anakit®

A commercial kit consisting of a multiple-use syringe of epinephrine (Adrenalin®) and chewable antihistamine tablets, with alcohol wipes and bandage. One-half the syringe amount (.3 ml) can be given before a twist is required to administer the second half of the injection. The standard adult dose required to treat anaphylactic shock due to severe allergic reactions from bee stings, etc., is .3 ml. AnaGuard® consists of the multiple injection syringe only. Use only on one person. See page 154.

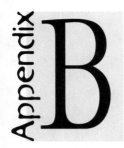

Appendix B

International Immunizations and Dosage Schedules

This section is of special relevance for the adventure traveler. Providing yourself with adequate time for proper pretrip medical travel consultation and immunization cannot be stressed too strongly. Not only must vaccine administration be sequenced properly but also adequate recovery time from possible reactions and time to acquire personal and prophylactic medications are essential.

Prior to any trip out of the country, call the U.S. Department of State Advisory Hotline at (202) 647–5225 for the latest information concerning political unrest. This number often includes health issues. Also call the Centers for Disease Control and Prevention International Travelers' Hotline at (404) 332–4559. Contact The International Association for Medical Assistance to Travellers (IAMAT) for their latest immunization recommendations and membership packet. Membership is free, but a donation is appreciated. In the United States their address is: 417 Center Street, Lewiston, NY 14092 (716) 754–4883; in Canada: 40 Regal Road, Guelph, Ontario, N1K 1B5 (519) 836–0102. For your convenience, information concerning routine childhood immunizations and links to current immunization information Web sites can be found at my Web site.

Cholera

Low levels of protection result from this vaccine. It is not recommended for inclusion in normal travel immunizations, but might be considered if high-risk exposure might occur in areas with active disease.

Primary immunization consists of two doses given subcutaneously or intramuscularly 1 week to 1 month or more apart. Booster injections are required every 6 months. Dosages are: children 6 months to 5 years, 0.2 ml; 5 to 10 years, 0.3 ml; over 10 years, 0.5 ml. Immunization is effective 6 days after receiving an injection—or immediately with boosters—but it provides approximately 30 to 50% protection for only 3 to 6 months.

This vaccine is generally not recommended for use in travelers due to its low level of effectiveness. If it is to be taken, a new dosage regimen of 0.2 ml given intradermal for persons age 5 and over causes less side effects and still fulfills potential government requirements for this vaccination. No government officially requires this vaccine, but some border crossing guards demand certification that you have had it. This problem is limited to a few African countries at this time. Side effects include pain at the injection site for 24 to 48 hours; possible local redness and swelling; fever, headache, malaise developing in most recipients and persisting for 1-2 days.

Hepatitis A (Infectious Hepatitis)

This vaccine should be obtained by all travelers going anywhere except Northern Europe, Canada, United States, Australia, and New Zealand.

Two vaccines are currently available in the United States: VAQTA by Merck & Company and Havrix by SmithKline Beecham Pharmaceuticals. The primary series for either must be completed 2 weeks prior to potential exposure. Neither is to be used in children less than 2 years of age. The adult dosing for both follows a similar schedule. One intramuscular injection of 1 ml of VAQTA 50 units or of 1 ml of Havrix 1440 EL.U. constitutes the basic immunization. VAQTA should be boosted in 6 months and Havrix in 6 to 12 months. For youngsters age 2 to 18 years the dose of Havrix is 720 EL.U./0.5 ml, followed by the same dose as a booster in 6 to 12 months. The VAQTA schedule for youngsters age 2 to 17 years is 25 U/0.5 ml, followed by the same dose as a booster in 6 to 19 months later. Re-immunization should be done in 3-year intervals for adults and children using the above doses of the respective vaccines.

A single dose of pooled immune globulin (10% solution) provides immediate protection against hepatitis A and can be used if the traveler is immediately departing and will be exposed prior to the 2 weeks required for the VAQTA or Havrix to form an adequate antibody response. The VAQTA or Havrix may be given simultaneously at different sites. Immune globulin must not be given at the same time as the measles, mumps, rubella (MMR) vaccine. It may be given at least 14 days after MMR or 6 weeks to 3 months (preferably 6 months) before MMR. There are no apparent problems in the administration of oral polio vaccine or yellow fever vaccine with or near immune globulin administration. Dosage depends upon body weight and length of time of required protection. At maximal doses it still must be repeated every 6 months for continued protection, but if VAQTA or Havrix has been obtained, the 3 month dose as shown on the following table is sufficient. Side effects are minimal other than rather mild possible pain at the injection site. Immune globulin must be given in the gluteal muscle, while VAQTA and Havrix are given in the deltoid muscle.

Immune Globulin Dosage*			Table B-1
weight	short term	long term	
	(< 3 months)	(>3 months)	
< 50 pounds	0.5 ml	1.0 ml	
50-100 pounds	1.0 ml	2.5 ml	
> 100 pounds	2.0 ml	5.0 ml	
	(repeat every 6 mos.)		

*Also called immune serum globulin and gamma globulin.

Hepatitis B (Serum Hepatitis)

Recommended as part of a standard immunization program regardless of travel.
Hepatitis B is most commonly spread by hypodermic usage, sexual contact, and blood transfusions. It has a very high prevalence in many areas of the world. Immunization is from a series of 1.0 ml IM injections of hepatitis B vaccine, called Recombivax HB® (Merck & Company) or Engerix-B (SmithKline Beecham). Either vaccine is usually given on day 0, 1 month, and 6 months. Special preparations of these vaccines and alternate schedules are used for children of various ages and for persons at very high risk, such as dialysis patients. Duration of protection and need for revaccination has not been defined. A blood test to determine adequate antibody response can be performed. If the antibody level falls below 10 SRUs, revaccination with 1.0 ml of vaccine should be considered. The injection must be given in the deltoid muscle. Side effects include: pain, inflammation at injection site; fatigue/weakness and low grade fever; nausea and diarrhea; sore throat and upper respiratory symptoms in 1% or slightly higher of recipients.

Influenza

Recommended for jet travelers during September through February, persons over the age of 65, and persons with chronic medical problems.
Vaccines are prepared that give 1 to 2 years of immunity for prevalent strains of influenza A or B. New strains are constantly arising that re-

quire new formulation to compensate for this "antigenic drift." Dosage is 0.5 ml IM in the deltoid muscle, given in the fall of the year. This vaccine is not required for routine travel, but may be suggested for the traveler heading into an epidemic area. Being confined on airplanes for long flights places you at high risk as the air breathed by everyone on the plane is recirculated. A booster of 0.5 ml must be given yearly. Fewer than one-third of recipients have local soreness around the injection for less than 2 days; fever, muscle ache, malaise can begin 6–12 hours after injection and last 1 or 2 days; persons with very severe egg allergy have increased risk of allergic reaction.

Japanese Encephalitis

To be given to travelers who will be exposed more than 3 weeks to rice farming or pig raising areas in Southeast Asia, Philippines, the southeastern Russian Federation, the Indian subcontinent, islands in the Torres Strait off the Australian mainland, and China or Korea during warm months.

Immunization requires 3 doses to be given at weekly intervals, with a booster dose at 12 to 18 months and at 4 year intervals thereafter, if risk continues. This vaccine is now available in the U.S. Reactions are infrequent in children, but occur in 0.6% of adult Western recipients. There have been no reports of demyelinating disease or encephalitis from the vaccine. Fever and local reactions develop in fewer than 10% of recipients. This vaccine should not be taken by pregnant women and persons with malignant diseases or other current illness.

Lyme Disease

For use by persons who are exposed to ticks in the Northeastern United States from Cape Cod, Massachusetts, to Maryland, Wisconsin/Minnesota border region, and Northern California.

LYMErix, a recombinant vaccine made by SmithKline Beecham, provides adequate protection with 3 doses. The compressed schedule of giving this vaccine at 0, 1, 2 months works as well as the FDA approved schedules which take longer. The series should be completed before the tick exposure season starts. It appears that a 1 dose booster should be given yearly.

Measles, Mumps, Rubella

Recommended as part of a standard immunization program regardless of travel.

One 0.5 ml dose given subcutaneously provides initial immunity. The MMR vaccine provides adequate protection against all three viral diseases, but each vaccine is available separately. May not be given if allergic to eggs or neomycin without special desensitization. This vaccine must be given at least 14 days prior to or 6 weeks to 3 months after immune serum globulin. All persons born after 1956 should receive a booster of measles containing vaccine to be considered immune. Side effects for these vaccines are as follows:

Measles: low grade fever (99° to 102° F, 37° to 39° C) may occur 5-12 days after injection, rarely a generalized rash develops; fever higher than 103° F (39.4° C) occurs less than 15% of the time. Allergy to chicken eggs and neomycin may cause an allergic reaction.

Mumps: burning and stinging of short duration at injection site; occasional mild fever; fever above 103° F is uncommon; allergic reactions at the injection site are extremely rare; swelling of the parotid salivary gland—low incidence; testicle inflammation is very rare; seizures, deafness, and encephalitis are very rare. Allergy to chicken eggs or feathers or to neomycin may cause an allergic reaction. Any active infection is reason to delay receiving this vaccine. Also any blood disorder, immune deficiency, or use of corticosteroid is a contraindication for vaccination.

Rubella: occasional moderate fever (101° to 102° F), less commonly high fever (over 103° F); burning at injection site; reactions are usually mild and transient, but include fever, rash, sore throat, nausea, vomiting, joint ache. Avoid giving to pregnant women, to persons with blood disorders, or to those receiving corticosteroid. Allergy to neomycin may cause an allergic reaction. Avoid giving if active illness is present.

Meningococcal Meningitis

Recommended for travelers to subSaharan Africa during the months of December to June. This vaccine is required for entry into Saudi Arabia during the period of the hajj. This vaccine should be considered for persons providing health care to refugee populations in Africa.

This vaccine need be used only under special circumstances (military personnel in the U.S. and persons traveling to those areas of the world indicated above where meningococcal infection is epidemic). The A/C/Y/W135 vaccine by Squibb-Connaught is given 0.5 ml subcutaneously. Duration of protection is unknown, but appears to be at least 3 years in those over 4 years of age. A booster shot of 0.5 ml should be given every 3 to 5 years based on new or continued exposure risk. There might be local redness at the injection site for 1 to 2 days. Reactions are uncommon and usually mild. This vaccine does not provide protection against the B serogroup of *N. Meningitidis,* which accounted for 28% of the U.S. (between 1994 and 1997) and some of the foreign outbreaks. A new vaccine for serogroup B is being tested now.

Plague

Only recommended for persons working in areas with active epidemics.

In most countries of Africa, Asia, and the Americas where plague is reported, the risk of exposure exists primarily in rural mountainous or upland areas. Adult immunization consists of 3 injections of 0.5 ml, 0.5 ml, and 0.2 ml (in that order) about 4 weeks apart and two boosters of 0.2 ml 6 months apart, then 1 dose every 1 to 2 years if needed. Local pain and inflammation is the most common side effect while generalized fever and illness is uncommon.

Pneumonia

Recommended for persons over 65 years of age and those with high risk, such as exposure to large numbers of people and those with chronic lung problems and debilitating conditions.

The vaccine against streptococcal (formerly called pneumococcal) pneumonia is given with one 0.5 ml IM injection, probably in the deltoid muscle. It should be boosted every 10 years. Local inflammation and pain at the injection site is relatively common, especially with the booster shot.

Poliomyelitis

A booster of inactivated polio vaccine is recommended for all persons born after 1956 traveling to Africa.

Injectable polio vaccine (IPV) is the vaccine of choice for all infants, children, and adolescents (up to their 18th birthday). The primary series is 3 doses, with dose 2 given at least 6 weeks after 1 and dose 3 given 8 to 12 months after dose 2. A supplemental dose is given to children at age 4 to 6 years. Anyone having a partial series may continue with the next dose(s), regardless of when the last dose was given. Unimmunized adults should be given the four full dose series of inactivated polio vaccine (IPV)(3 doses given at 1 to 2 month intervals, followed by a 4th dose 6 to 12 months after the 3rd dose), if time allows, or a minimum of 2 doses of IPV given a month apart. If less than a month remains prior to departure, the administration of a single dose of trivalent oral polio vaccine (OPV) may be justified in case of potential high risk of exposure to wild polio virus and the more rapid protective effect of OPV.

The good news is that there has been a significant decrease in wild strains of polio in the past few years, due to the massive world immunization program. There are very slight chances of adverse reactions with either polio vaccine. Vaccine associate disease in 1 per (oral) 8.7 million doses; disease in contacts incidence is 1 per 5.1 million doses. Any active infection is reason to delay receiving this vaccine. Also any blood disorder, immune deficiency, or use of corticosteroid is a contraindication for vaccination. No vaccine-associated disease reported with the injectable vaccine, although there is a slight chance of allergy in people sensitive to cow serum, neomycin, and streptomycin.

Rabies

Recommended if traveling in remote areas of Iraq, Iran, and Central Africa.

A pre-exposure regimen of rabies vaccine is appropriate for persons routinely exposed to potential rabid animals—including skunks, foxes, raccoons, and bats. It does not eliminate the need for additional therapy after rabies exposure, but simplifies post-exposure therapy by eliminating the requirement for rabies immune globulin (RIG) and by decreasing the number of doses of vaccine required. Prevention with human diploid cell vaccine (HDCV) is 3 doses given 1.0 ml IM in the deltoid muscle on days 0, 7, and 21 or 28. A new dosage of 0.1 ml intradermally given on the same dosage schedule also seems effective for prophylaxis. Caution should be taken to avoid taking chloroquine for malaria prophylaxis while receiving rabies immunization as it has been shown to reduce the antibody response.

Post-exposure immunization for those previously immunized is 2 doses (1 ml each) on days 0 and 3, with no RIG. If no prior immunization, give RIG 20 IU/kg (injecting as much as possible into and around the bite site and and any additional IM at a site distant from the HDCV injection site) and 5 doses (1 ml each) of HDCV on days 0, 3, 7, 14, and 28. These injections must be given in the deltoid muscle as 2 incidents of failure of post-exposure immunization with RIG and HDCV have occurred when these injections were given in the gluteal muscle.

To determine if a booster is needed, obtain antibody testing every two years. There is a very low incidence of side effect with the new diploid cell vaccine; some local irritation possible and occasional muscle ache and headache. In persons receiving a booster shot up to 6% may have hives, lymph node enlargement, and fever.

Tetanus–Diphtheria

Recommended as part of a standard immunization program regardless of travel.
Everyone should have a tetanus booster every 10 years; 5 years for
puncture wounds, bites, and other contaminated wounds. This vaccine is
so effective, a booster more often than every 10 years is probably not required. Dosage is 0.5 ml of dT vaccine given IM. A different vaccine is
used for children. Infants receive a special diphtheria–tetanus–pertussis
(DTP) vaccine, which is also a different formulation than that used for
children. Family physicians, pediatricians, and travel medicine clinics
generally have all three vaccines in stock at all times. Both adults' and
children's vaccines should be given with diphtheria toxoid in combination. Infants should follow the routine pediatric immunization schedule
with diphtheria–tetanus–pertussis–Hib combination vaccine. A local reaction at injection site is possible; fever may occur; severe allergic reactions are rare.

Typhoid

*Recommended for travelers outside of the United States, northern Europe,
Australia, and New Zealand.*
Three typhoid vaccines are available in the United States. The oldest,
Typhoid USP is the least expensive, but requires 2 doses given subcutaneously at an interval of 4 or more weeks. A compressed schedule of 3
doses at weekly intervals may also be used. Both regimens provide approximately 70% effectiveness. Booster requirement for the injectable
vaccine is 0.5 ml subcutaneously (or 0.1 ml intradermal) every 3 years.
Local pain at the injection site occurs in most recipients; fever, lethargy,
headache may last for 1 to 2 days. This vaccine may be given to pregnant women. Allergy to phenol may cause an allergic reaction. The side
effects of this vaccine, particularly severe pain at the injection site, are
much higher than with the two new vaccines now available.

A new high potency oral vaccine became available in 1990 that provides at least 80% effective protection and has considerably fewer side
effects than the USP vaccine. Immunization is with 1 capsule of the live
attenuated Ty21a vaccine [Vivotif® (Berna) made by the Swiss Serum
and Vaccine Institute], taken every other day for four doses (day 0, 2, 4,
6). Booster requirements for the oral vaccine have not been determined
but efficacy has been shown to persist at least 5 years. Therefore, an adequate booster will be achieved by repeating the 4 capsule every-other-
day regime every 5 years.

A new injectable vaccine produced by Pasteur Mérieux Sérums & Vaccins and distributed in the U.S. by Connaught is the Typhim Vi polysaccharide vaccine. Studies show a four-fold increase in antibody protection in 88 to 96% of recipients. Efficacy studies have demonstrated protection rates from disease during exposure of 55%. Immunization dosage is a single .5 ml injection given IM. A booster is recommended using a single .5 ml injection every 2 years.

Yellow Fever

Immunization is required for travel to many countries in South America, Africa, and Asia.

The immunization consists of one 0.5 ml injection, which confers immunity for 10 years. It is available only at designated Yellow Fever Vaccination Centers (check your County or State Board of Health for the nearest facility). The booster dose is the same amount every 10 years. Approximately 5 to 10% of recipients experience headache, lethargy, muscle ache, and fever, which occurs 5 to 10 days after vaccination. This immunization must be recorded on an International Certificate of Immunization and will not be considered valid for 10 days from the time of receipt.

Clinical Reference Index